ALARYNGEAL
SPEECH REHABILITATION

To Willie Diedrich, who conducted research with laryngectomees that has withstood the test of time; Marshall Duguay, who has been a teacher of clinicians and an advocate for laryngectomized patients; and Jim Shanks, who has traveled the world to promote alaryngeal speech rehabilitation.

> Cover portrait of *(left to right)* Jim Shanks, Marshall Duguay, and Willie Diedrich by John Wilson of Austin, Texas.

FOR CLINICIANS BY CLINICIANS
Harris Winitz, Series Editor

This book, *Alaryngeal Speech Rehabilitation,* is the fifth volume in the For Clinicians by Clinicians series of texts on the diagnosis and clinical management of speech, language, and voice disorders. Each text provides a contemporary perspective on one major disorder or clinical area and is designed for use in clinical methodology courses and continuing education programs. Authors have been selected who represent a broad spectrum of clinical interests and theoretical positions and who hold the common belief that their viewpoints, experiences, and successes should be shared in order to provide a forum for clinicians by clinicians.

Volumes already published in this series are *Treating Language Disorders, Treating Articulation Disorders, Case Studies in Aphasia Rehabilitation, Treating Cerebral Palsy,* and *Treating Disordered Speech Motor Control.*

ALARYNGEAL SPEECH REHABILITATION

For Clinicians by Clinicians

Edited by
Shirley J. Salmon and Kay H. Mount

pro·ed
8700 Shoal Creek Boulevard
Austin, Texas 78758

Printed in the United States of America

Library of Congress Cataloging-in-Publication Data

Alaryngeal speech rehabilitation / edited by Shirley Salmon and Kay
   Mount.
      p.   cm.—(For clinicians by clinicians)
   Includes bibliographical references.
   ISBN 0-89079-415-4
   1. Laryngectomees—Rehabilitation. 2. Speech, Alaryngeal.
I. Salmon, Shirley J. II. Mount, Kay. III. Series.
   [DNLM: 1. Laryngectomy—rehabilitation. 2. Speech, Alaryngeal.
WV 540 A323]
RF540.A43   1991
617.5′3301—dc20
DNLM/DLC   90-9164
for Library of Congress   CIP

pro·ed
8700 Shoal Creek Boulevard
Austin, Texas 78758

1 2 3 4 5 6 7 8 9 10   95 94 93 92 91

Contents

Contributors

Zilpha T. Bosone, PhD
Audiology and Speech Pathology
  Service (126)
Veterans Administration Medical
  Center
50 Irving Street, NW
Washington, DC 20422

Mary A. Carpenter, PhD
Hearing and Speech Department
3031 H. C. Miller Building
University of Kansas Medical
  Center
Rainbow Boulevard at 39th Street
Kansas City, KS 66103

William M. Diedrich, PhD
Hearing and Speech Department
3031 H. C. Miller Building
University of Kansas Medical
  Center
Rainbow Boulevard at 39th Street
Kansas City, KS 66103

Marshall J. Duguay, PhD
Speech–Language Pathology
State University at Buffalo
1300 Elmwood Avenue
Buffalo, NY 14222

Stuart I. Gilmore, PhD
Department of Speech and Hearing
  Sciences
Humboldt State University
Arcata, CA 95521-4957

Samuel K. Haroldson, MA
Department of Communication
  Disorders
115 Shevlin Hall
University of Minnesota
164 Pillsbury Drive, SE
Minneapolis, MN 55455

Robert L. Keith, MA
Speech Pathology
Department of Neurology
Mayo Clinic
Rochester, MN 55905

Jay W. Lerman, PhD
Department of Communication
  Sciences
Box U-85
University of Connecticut
850 Bolton Road
Storrs, CT 06268

Stanley J. Martinkosky, PhD
Hearing and Speech Center
North Carolina Memorial Hospital
Chapel Hill, NC 27514

Kay H. Mount, PhD
Beggs Telephone Company, Inc.
5th and Choctaw
P.O. Box 749
Beggs, OK 74421

Shirley J. Salmon, PhD
Audiology and Speech Pathology
  (126)
Veterans Administration Medical
  Center
4801 Linwood Boulevard
Kansas City, MO 64128

James C. Shanks, PhD
Speech Pathology Services
Department of Otolaryngology–
  Head and Neck Surgery
Indiana University School of
  Medicine
702 Barnhill Drive, Suite A56
Indianapolis, IN 46223

Martha Strasser
8021 Icking
Talberg 26
Federal Republic of Germany

Preface

When presented with the opportunity to edit a text on alaryngeal speech, we wondered whether another book about laryngectomee rehabilitation would be worthwhile. We discussed whether the available information was meeting the need for which it was intended, and concluded that it was not. Our work with graduate students and clinicians had shown us that often they had only rudimentary knowledge about methods of alaryngeal speech and even less knowledge about how to proceed with solving treatment problems.

The clinician's ability to integrate information seemed to be the missing link in providing effective treatment. Much of the information about laryngectomees apparently had been presented to students and clinicians in a factual manner with the implied assumption that professionals would relate it intuitively to the clinical process. For whatever reasons, most professionals have not done so. We decided that a more effective approach might be to present information in a tutorial fashion so that speech–language pathologists could understand the thought processes underlying treatment. The contributing authors were asked to imagine they were tutoring an individual and teaching that person what to do, when to do it, and why. Meeting such a challenge has been difficult, and we appreciate the efforts of the contributors who spent so much time refining their chapters. We are proud of the small part we have played in shaping this book. Our task was made easier because all of the contributors are practicing clinicians who are well known for their knowledge, clinical or research skills, ability to teach, and love of working with laryngectomees.

The contributors have written about many issues related to rehabilitation of laryngectomees. In the first chapter, Diedrich compares the anatomy and physiology of laryngeal and alaryngeal individuals and provides a basis for understanding the morphology of esophageal speech. In chapter 2, Lerman addresses artificial larynx speech and discusses its value even as an aid to learning esophageal speech. Chapters 3, 4, and 5 focus on esophageal speech training. Duguay describes the initial phases of treatment; Haroldson writes about an ongoing refinement program; and Salmon and Mount discuss the philosophical and pragmatic aspects of group therapy. Martinkosky in chapter 6 and Bosone in chapter 7 thoroughly cover treatment procedures appropriate for patients undergoing the Singer–Blom voice restoration procedure. Carpenter gives careful consideration to perceptual judgments of alaryngeal speech in chapter 8. She examines the pros and cons of using judgments to influence treatment decisions. In chapter 9, Gilmore explores physical, social, occupational, and psychological causes of failure in esophageal speech acquisition and suggests prevention programs. Strasser, who was married to a laryngectomee for many years, presents unique material in chapter 10 regarding concerns common to spouses of all laryngectomized patients. In chapter 11, Shanks shares a wealth of material about laryngectomees' compensatory behaviors. Most of this material has not been presented previously and is the accumulation of his many years of clinical experience. In the concluding chapter, Keith explains how to organize and conduct a successful conference that addresses alaryngeal speech rehabilitation.

We hope that as students and clinicians read this text, they will better understand the essence of the treatment process, and that this understanding will encourage them, through their own practice, to continue the work of the contributing authors. We are particularly grateful for the contributions of Diedrich, Duguay, Shanks, and Strasser who have retired this year.

CHAPTER 1

Anatomy and Physiology of Esophageal Speech

William M. Diedrich

Diedrich provides a comprehensive comparison of the anatomy and physiology of laryngeal and alaryngeal individuals. Thus, he provides a basis for understanding the complexity of esophageal speech communication and lays the foundation for the chapters that follow.

Study Questions

1. *Why is an understanding of the pharyngoesophageal segment anatomy and physiology critical to the teaching of esophageal voice?*

2. *Since pulmonary air is no longer used for purposes of phonation, what relevance does respiratory function have in the development of esophageal voice?*

3. *Despite the limited capacity of the esophagus, how can the duration of esophageal voice be increased?*

LARYNGEAL EXTIRPATION

A laryngectomy is the surgical removal of the larynx. In other surgical procedures, such as hemilaryngectomy, partial laryngectomy, and supraglottic laryngectomy, parts of the larynx are removed. Although patients undergoing these latter procedures also may require the skills of a speech clinician, the discussion in this chapter is limited to total laryngectomy and the anatomy and physiology of esophageal speech. Other forms of postlaryngectomy *(alaryngeal)* speech are discussed in the chapters that follow.

The normal vocal tract includes the lips, teeth, oral cavity, velum, pharynx, and larynx. When a laryngectomy is performed, the larynx is removed (including the hyoid bone) and the top of the trachea is sewn to the base of the neck where a permanent opening *(tracheostoma)* is created into the respiratory tract (Figure 1.1). After the larynx is removed, respiration takes place through the tracheostoma rather than the nose.

Following a laryngectomy, the complex valvular mechanism of the larynx which permits deglutition or respiration is no longer present. The hypopharynx is sewn to the upper esophagus so that food and liquids go directly to the esophagus without interfering with respiration (Figure 1.1). Because the hypopharynx—the common cavity for food and respiration—has been permanently altered by the laryngectomy, respiration is directed through the tracheostoma and deglutition in the hypopharynx no longer endangers the airway (Figure 1.2).

The fully clothed laryngectomee appears to the casual observer as normal as any person. As with a stutterer or deaf person, however, when a laryngectomee speaks, the listener becomes aware of a difference. The laryngectomee, in addition to having a "speech disorder," has profound adjustments in such physiological aspects of everyday living as breathing, coughing, crying, laughing, sucking through a straw, swimming, tasting, smelling, blowing the nose, and sometimes lifting heavy objects (discussed in chapter 11).

When the normal respiratory supply for speech has been altered and the laryngeal mechanism removed, can the laryngectomee learn to talk again? The answer is yes. If successfully acquired, esophageal speech seems simple and sounds surprisingly intelligible. Air is taken into the esophagus and expelled upward past tissues located in the pharyngoesophageal segment. When these tissues are set into vibration, sound is produced and articulated into fluent speech. Although esophageal speech has been referenced in the literature for more than 100 years, many aspects of this form of communication remain unclear. The following sections describe the anatomy and physiology necessary for

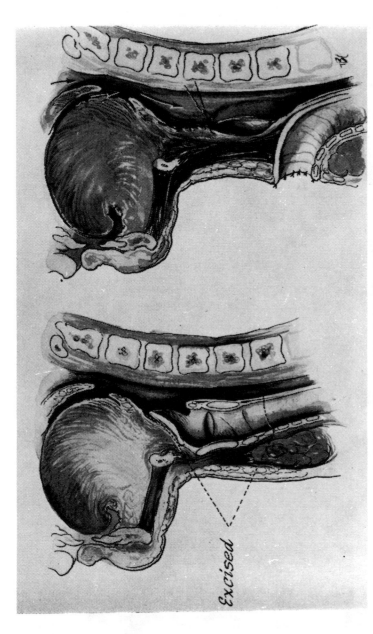

Figure 1.1. Total laryngectomy. On the left is a half section of the head and neck demonstrating the preoperative arrangement of the mouth, pharynx, and larynx. On the right is the change in arrangement after removal of the larynx. The severed end of the trachea has been brought forward and sutured to a hole in the skin of the neck. The hiatus created in the pharynx by removal of the larynx is being closed with sutures. From *Speech Rehabilitation of the Laryngectomized* (2nd ed., p. 28) by J. Snidecor and Others, 1969, Springfield, IL: Charles C. Thomas. Reprinted by permission.

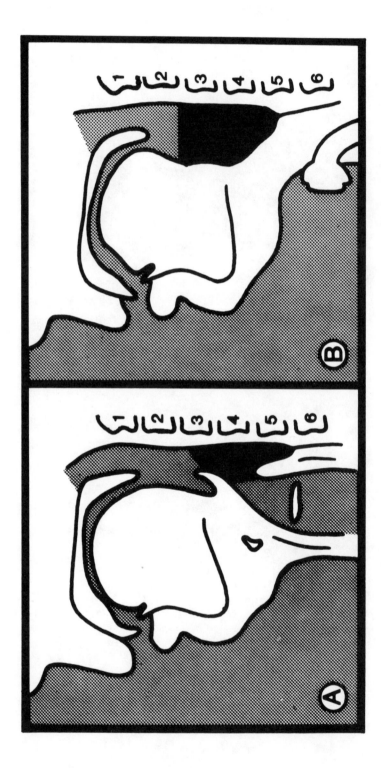

Figure 1.2. Preoperative and postoperative hyphopharynx. The radiographs illustrate (A) the hypopharynx (blackened area) as a common cavity for respiration and deglutition before laryngectomy and (B) the hypopharynx separated for respiration and deglutition after laryngectomy. In esophageal speakers, the hypopharynx is shared for esophageal air intake and air expulsion, as well as for deglutition.

esophageal speech. What appears to be a relatively simple communicative function is in fact quite complex.

NORMAL FUNCTION OF THE PHARYNGOESOPHAGEAL SEGMENT

Muscle Fibers

Because the fibers of the inferior pharyngeal constrictor, cricopharyngeus, and upper esophagus are blended, the area composed of all three sets of fibers is referred to commonly as the pharyngoesophageal (PE) segment, sphincter, or junction. The inferior pharyngeal constrictor comprises oblique fibers which attach posteriorly to the anterior of the laryngeal structures. The fibers of the inferior pharyngeal constrictor merge with the cricopharyngeus muscle, which consists of circular fibers attached anteriorly to the cricoid cartilage, forming a U-shaped sling. The inferior fibers of the cricopharyngeus muscle join the circular fibers of the upper esophagus (Zaino, Jacobson, Lepow, & Ozturk, 1970). The esophagus is composed of two layers of tissue: the inner layer is circular and the outer layer is longitudinal (Figure 1.3). The cervical upper esophagus is composed of striated muscle fibers, the lower third is smooth involuntary muscle, and the thoracic middle third consists of both smooth and striated muscle fibers (Payne & Olsen, 1974). This point is important to remember because striated muscle is under control of the cortex and, presumably, under conscious voluntary control. Smooth muscle is under control of the autonomic nervous system, and thus is involuntary.

Neural Innervation

The PE segment appears to be innervated by the nucleus ambiguus and the dorsal vagal nucleus, carried by the X cranial nerve and, to a lesser extent, the IX and XI cranial nerves (Inglefinger, 1958). Decroix, Libersa, and Lattard (1958) and Storchi and Micheli-Pellegrini (1959) stated that branches of the recurrent laryngeal nerve are directed to the PE segment. Zaino et al. (1970) believed that the cricopharyngeus is under voluntary control but that the upper esophageal sphincter is "innervated by both the central and the sympathetic system in spite of its striated muscle" (p. 71). In addition, Ekberg (1986) stated:

> The somatic efferent motor control from the nucleus ambiguus via the tenth and eleventh cranial nerves is agreed, whereas consensus is lacking about the contribution of sympathetic and para-sympathetic innervation. Other aspects of innervation of the [PE] segment are poorly understood. (p. 877)

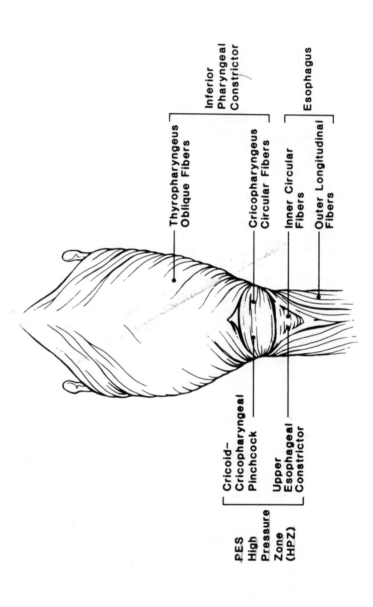

Figure 1.3. The pharyngoesophageal sphincter (PES) high pressure zone (HPZ). The upper component is the cricoid–cricopharyngeus pinchcock and the lower component is the upper esophageal constrictor. Adapted from "Upper Esophageal Sphincter: Pre- and Post-laryngectomy—A Normative Study" by G. A. Gates, 1980, *Laryngoscope, 90,* p. 455. Adapted by permission of *Laryngoscope,* St. Louis, MO. Reprinted by permission.

Physiology

The PE segment has been generically called the upper esophageal sphincter (Gerhardt, Hewett, Moeschberger, Shuck, & Winship, 1980; Welch, Gates, Luckmann, Ricks & Drake, 1979; Welch, Luckmann, Ricks, Drake, & Gates, 1979). Welch, Gates, et al. (1979) and Welch, Luckmann, et al. (1979) evaluated pressures within the PE segment with intraluminal catheters, providing *manometric* data. When computer analyzed and projected three-dimensionally, the data demonstrated upper and lower zones of constriction within the PE segment. Gates (1980) suggested that the PE segment be described as the pharyngo-esophageal sphincter high pressure zone (PES-HPZ). The cricoid–cricopharyngeus pinchcock represents the upper component, and the upper esophageal constrictor, or upper esophageal sphincter, represents the lower component (see Figure 1.3). Both of these pressure components would be within the traditionally described PE segment or the so-called high pressure zone (HPZ).

The purpose for this HPZ appears to be twofold. First, the PE segment tonic closure prevents aerophagia during normal respiration; that is, during normal pulmonary inspiration, atmospheric air is directed into the larynx, trachea, and lungs, and the PE sphincter prevents air from being insufflated into the esophagus. Second, the HPZ prevents gastric reflux from the esophagus into the hypopharynx, larynx, and airway.

During deglutition and belching, the normal PE segment closure must be inhibited and the HPZ must temporarily relax. As a bolus of food enters the hypopharynx, the laryngeal valves close, the larynx is elevated upward and forward, and the HPZ markedly decreases in constriction to permit peristalsis to propel the bolus through the PE segment. Inglefinger (1958) assumed that a reflex inhibitory wave relaxes the PE segment. However, the upward and forward elevation of the larynx also may provide a mechanical opening of the cricopharyngeal pinchcock (Gates, 1980). The opening of the lower component of the HPZ, the upper esophageal sphincter, is presumably on a neural basis. When gas is generated in the stomach and a belch is induced, pressure is decreased in the HPZ; that is, when gas from the stomach enters and dilates the esophagus, a concomitant decrease in pressure occurs as the gas continues to pass upward through the PE segment to produce a belch (Kahrilas et al., 1986).

The neural control of the PE segment is important to an understanding of the acquisition of esophageal speech. Teaching someone how to control the constriction of the PE segment is paramount in teaching that person to learn esophageal speech.

THE PHARYNGOESOPHAGEAL SEGMENT
AFTER LARYNGECTOMY

During surgical removal of the larynx, the anterior fibers of the inferior pharyngeal constrictor which were attached to the larynx and the anterior fibers of the cricopharyngeus which were attached to the cricoid cartilage must be sutured. Whether a circular ring of muscle tissue is ever accomplished has been seriously questioned (Dey & Kirchner, 1961). The sutured tissue must be leakproof so that food and liquid can be swallowed into the hypopharynx and then into the esophagus (see Figures 1.1 and 1.2).

The PE segment may look and function quite differently before and after the laryngectomy. The morphology and function of the PE segment was a primary focus of study by Diedrich and Youngstrom (1966). They observed the PE segment to have a variety of shapes with tissue on the ventral and dorsal side of the PE lumen. Six subjects had double segments. No relation between morphology and speech skill was observed (for examples of different PE morphology, see chapter 3). Correlations of speech skill with the PE segment axial length during phonation were nonsignificant. Many investigators have postulated that the cricopharyngeus was the only structure that makes a suitable pseudolarynx. Diedrich and Youngstrom concluded that "probably fibers from the inferior constrictor and the superior esophageal sphincter, as well as the cricopharyngeus muscle, compose the neoglottis" (p. 59). In addition, some patients had no obvious PE segment constriction, others had double segments, and some had neoglottises higher than the typical placement at the level of the fifth or sixth cervical vertebra.

Another predictor of PE segment function is deglutition. Patients who continue to have postoperative swallowing difficulties (dysphagia) reportedly have not learned esophageal speech (Gates, Ryan, Cantu, & Hearne, 1982; Volin, 1980). In Gates et al.'s study, none of the patients who needed dilation for stricture of the PE segment developed esophageal speech.

Results conflict regarding the amount of pressure necessary in the HPZ for successful esophageal sound. Manometric studies of the HPZ have produced pressure readings that average 121 mm Hg before surgery and 50 mm Hg after surgery (Welch, Luckmann, et al., 1979). These investigators found no difference in the PE-HPZ in patients who learned esophageal speech and those who did not acquire esophageal speech. These results confirmed earlier studies (Dey & Kirchner, 1961), but are in contrast to Winans, Reichbach, and Waldrop's (1974) study in which sphincter pressure was found to be lower in patients who acquired fluent esophageal speech and higher in those who did not develop esophageal speech.

Bosone-Crouch (1974) studied intraluminal pressure measures 1 cm below the PE segment, within the PE segment, and 1 cm above the PE segment during three tasks: resting, swallowing, and esophageal phonation of /a/. Phonation was evaluated on two dimensions: "goodness" and duration. During the phonation task, pressure measures accounted for 33% of the variance for both goodness ratings and maximum duration of phonation. Similar pressure measures were found in the best and poorest phonators. Bosone-Crouch concluded that PE segment area pressures can be used neither to predict goodness or maximum duration of phonation, nor to predict which PE segments are "too loose" or "too tight."

The implication of the PE-HPZ for speech training is that for acquisition of successful esophageal speech, the laryngectomee must learn to take air into the esophagus easily and quickly and, conversely, to expel the air from the esophagus into the oral cavity. If resistance in the PE-HPZ is so high that either maneuver is prevented, then esophageal voice will fail to occur.

ESOPHAGEAL AIR SUPPLY

In laryngeal speakers the duration and intensity of the vocal tone is dependent not only upon the vibrator (size, shape, elasticity, density, etc., of the vocal cords), but also upon the pulmonary air supply. Persons with emphysema, or other limits on respiratory performance, do not have good vocal duration or intensity. In learning esophageal speech, the laryngectomee is dependent upon the esophageal reservoir for containing the air used in speech. Obviously, the esophagus capacity is small compared with that of the lungs. The capacity of the esophagus is considered to range from 40 to 80 cc (van den Berg & Moolenaar-Bijl, 1959). For comparison, the vital capacity of lungs in healthy adults ranges from 2,200 to 4,690 cc (Loudon, Lee, & Holcomb, 1988). Snidecor and Isshiki (1965a) found that for 51 words, volume ranged from 372 to 1,115 cc (median of 935 cc) for 6 esophageal speakers, compared with an average of 3,020 cc for laryngeal speakers. The volume of air per syllable during continuous speech was 12.4 to 15.9 cc in 6 esophageal speakers and averaged 43.1 cc per syllable for laryngeal speakers.

Airflow rates during exsufflation are important elements of esophageal voice. These rates are determined by the volume of air trapped in the esophagus, the pressure developed in the esophagus on exsufflation, and the resistance from the PE segment (vibrator). These principles are similar to those observed in laryngeal voice production.

AIR INTAKE

Injection and inhalation are the two basic methods for air intake into the esophagus. In a study of 27 esophageal speakers, Diedrich and Youngstrom (1966) found 20 to be injectors and 7 to be inhalers.

The injection process is accomplished through the use of the tongue as a piston in an airtight cylinder. The tongue blade is in contact with the hard and soft palate to prevent the anterior flow of air. The tongue makes a dorsad (i.e., backward) motion toward the pharyngeal wall. Sometimes the tongue contacts the pharynx and sometimes it does not (Diedrich & Youngstrom, 1966). Velopharyngeal closure must always be present. Otherwise, the air in the mouth which is being compressed by the backward motion of the tongue will be forced into the nasal cavities and out the nares instead of being forced into the hypopharynx, past the PE segment, and into the esophagus. If the tonic closure of the PE segment is stronger than the air compressed by the tongue, the air will not enter the esophagus and true esophageal tone will not be possible. Frequently, air compressed in the hypopharynx will be pressed upward between the tongue and the pharyngeal wall, producing a lingual–pharyngeal friction noise. This sound can be developed into what is known as pharyngeal speech (because the air reservoir in this case is the hypopharynx). The clinician must be alert to this phenomenon and develop auditory discrimination to distinguish pharyngeal and esophageal sounds. A pharyngeal sound can be made by forcing the tongue against the posterior pharyngeal wall and producing a modified /k/ sound. The tone produced should be contrasted with the familiar belch-like (esophageal) sound which comes from gas generated in the stomach. Pharyngeal sounds should be avoided, and the clinician must not reinforce the pharyngeal tone in the belief that it is an esophageal tone.

In the inhalation method, the PE segment must be relaxed (open) sufficiently for atmospheric air pressure in the oral cavity and hypopharynx to fill the partial vacuum in the esophagus. The esophagus is normally a collapsed muscular tube which contains a negative amount of air pressure in contrast to positive atmospheric air pressure. The intraesophageal air pressure at rest is -4 to -7 mm Hg below atmospheric pressure (Inglefinger, 1958; Kramer, Atkinson, Wyman, & Inglefinger, 1957).

During inhalation the tongue does not occlude the oral cavity and a dorsad movement of the posterior tongue is not visible as in injection. Usually the lips are open and the velopharyngeal port is closed (Diedrich & Youngstrom, 1966). A patent airway is maintained between the lips and the PE junction, enabling atmospheric air pressure (approximately

14 psi at sea level) to insufflate the partial vacuum in the esophagus. Some patients move the air through the nose instead of through the mouth, in which case the velopharyngeal mechanism must remain open to enable the atmospheric air pressure to flow from the nasal cavities into the hypopharynx and then into the esophagus.

This normal respiratory effect on esophageal air pressure works to the advantage of the inhaler. During normal pulmonary inhalation, the negative pressure in the esophagus at rest (-4 to -7 mm Hg) may be increased to -10 to -15 mm Hg (Atkinson, Kramer, Wyman, & Inglefinger, 1957). The increased partial vacuum (negative pressure) results in a higher potential for positive atmospheric air pressure to be pulled (sucked) into the esophagus. Critical to this whole process is the amount of sphincteric contraction of the PE segment. The PE segment tissues must relax sufficiently to permit the exchange of air from the vocal tract into the esophagus.

HOW IS AIR DISCHARGED FROM THE ESOPHAGUS?

Less information is available about this particular stage of esophageal speech than any other.

> If the understanding of the mechanisms of air intake is not clear and seems complex, the dynamics of air expulsion are still more enigmatic. There are several problems to be resolved, including the morphology and physiology of the esophagus, its cephalad and caudad sphincters, the position of the esophagus within the chest cavity, and the effect on the esophagus of interpulmonary pressure changes, diaphragmatic tension, stomach pressures, and abdominal contractions. (Diedrich, 1968, p. 308)

Normal forced pulmonary expiration is characterized by elastic recoil of the lungs, collapse of the thorax, and contraction of abdominal–intercostal muscles (Hixon, 1973). A similar respiratory maneuver is believed to help force air out of the esophagus. Increased pulmonary and intrathoracic exhalation pressure, against the adjoining inflated esophagus, pushes the air upward out of the esophagus. Why "upward" and not "downward" into the stomach? As long as the lower esophageal sphincter (between the esophagus and the stomach) exerts a higher pressure (is closed tighter) than the PE segment tonic closure, then intrathoracic–abdominal pressure against the esophagus will compress the air in an upward direction, setting into vibration the PE segment. Van den Berg, Moolenaar-Bijl, and Damsté (1958) speculated that with increased intrathoracic pressure, the esophagus may protrude between the tracheal rings, resulting in marked increase in the esophageal pressure. At the same time, they observed no increase in airflow from the lungs.

The interesting report of Kahrilas et al. (1986) may have importance here. In their study, distention of the esophagus during a belch resulted in a decrease in pressure of the HPZ of the upper esophageal sphincter and not in the lower esophageal sphincter (between esophagus and stomach). This phenomenon needs to be studied to determine whether similar reductions in the HPZ occur in persons who use esophageal speech.

RESPIRATORY FUNCTION AND ESOPHAGEAL SPEECH

Pulmonary respiration is indispensable in normal speech: for phonation to occur, a flow of air is needed to vibrate the vocal cords. After laryngectomy, the pulmonary air supply has been diverted through the tracheostoma and is not used for esophageal speech (Figure 1.1). However, intrathoracic pressures that are developed during pulmonary respiration seem to influence esophageal speech.

As previously mentioned, the two basic ways to put air into the esophagus are inhalation and injection. For the inhaler, pulmonary inspiration and esophageal insufflation must be synchronized. As noted earlier, when respiratory inspiration occurs, negative pressures in the esophagus simultaneously increase (from -4 to -7 mm Hg to -15 to -20 mm Hg). When the inhaler relaxes the tonic PE segment, atmospheric air fills the esophagus during pulmonary inspiration. When pulmonary expiration occurs, positive pressures of 25 mm Hg may be recorded in the esophagus during phonation (Dey & Kirchner, 1961). Consequently, the exhalation of pulmonary air is viewed as one factor that contributes to the expulsion of esophageal air, as described in the previous section. In other words, pulmonary air and esophageal air usually enter and exit in a synchronous fashion.

Injection through pistonlike pumping action of the tongue generally takes place in synchrony with respiration. During a phrase utterance, the injector tends to coordinate pulmonary inhalation with esophageal injection at the beginning of a phrase utterance. Pulmonary exhalation and esophageal phonation likewise are usually synchronous. Although synchrony is common with both injectors and inhalers, asynchrony of the pulmonary and esophageal systems has been recorded (Isshiki & Snidecor, 1965).

The inexperienced clinician and the newly laryngectomized patient need to be aware that during the patient's early stages of acquiring speech, two behaviors associated with respiration—coughing and hyperventilation—may occur. Coughing can occur as a result of practicing air intake/expulsion. Forcing pulmonary air through the trachea may irritate the mucous lining of the trachea and cause the patient to cough.

Continued coughing may lead to bleeding, and expectoration of the blood can alarm the patient. The clinician might do one of two things after explaining to the patient what happened: (a) Terminate practice of esophageal speech training at that point and resume later, or (b) ask the patient to reduce the force of pulmonary air expulsion while attempting esophageal phonation, which not only reduces the risk of tracheal irritation, but also reduces stoma noise.

Hyperventilation—the deep and rapid exchange of pulmonary air—may result in dizziness in the early stages of esophageal speech training. Patients should be cautioned about this lightheadedness so that they will know what to expect while practicing esophageal speech. Hyperventilation is more apt to occur in patients who are practicing the inhalation rather than the injection technique of air intake. To alleviate this condition, (a) reduce the pulmonary effort of air intake and air expulsion, and (b) reduce the frequency of trials within a specified time period.

OTHER ANATOMIC/PHYSIOLOGIC CONSIDERATIONS

Production of esophageal sound is simply the beginning of a laryngectomee's long road to recovery of successful communication. Other important objectives include avoidance of nonesophageal sounds, intelligible articulation, and increased duration and intensity of the tone.

Variations in Alaryngeal Phonation (Buccal and Pharyngeal Speech)

Buccal and pharyngeal sounds are nonesophageal sounds that should be avoided. *Buccal* speech refers to friction noises made by the tongue in a variety of positions in the oral cavity or by air squeezed between the cheeks and the alveolar ridge. *Pharyngeal* speech refers to sounds made primarily in the back of the mouth (oropharynx and hypopharynx) produced by the tongue pressed against the pillar of fauces, hard and soft palate, or posterior pharyngeal wall. Attempts at phonation that produce buccal or pharyngeal sounds should be immediately discouraged. Pharyngeal sounds are particularly insidious, and the clinician needs to teach the patient to make the distinction between pharyngeal and esophageal sounds.

In addition to buccal and pharyngeal sounds, a patient may produce a pharyngeal-like tone by vibrating a PE segment high in the hypopharynx at the level of the second or third cervical vertebra rather than the fifth or sixth cervical vertebra (Damsté, Van den Berg, & Moolenaar-Bijl, 1956; Diedrich & Youngstrom, 1966). The air supply may be deep in the hypopharynx at cervical vertebra 4 or 5 and above the lip of the esophagus. The relatively high placement of the neoglottis produces a sound that is perceived as high in pitch, weak in intensity, and thin in quality. The clinician should teach the patient to distinguish this higher pitched tone from the lower pitched tone associated with a belch. The patient should focus on producing sounds that are belchlike in pitch and quality. The goal is for the air reservoir to become located in the esophagus.

As noted earlier, PE segment tonicity is reduced following the laryngectomy. Some authors contend that little or no pressure is necessary for phonation to take place (e.g., Dey & Kirchner, 1961). However, a certain minimum approximation is required or no phonation (or only weak and brief duration of sound) will take place. Diedrich and Youngstrom (1966, pp. 133ff) described in detail a case study supporting this statement. Digital compression or the use of a neckband that applies pressure in the PE segment area often results in striking improvement in the quality of esophageal voice.

On the other hand, PE segment resistance may be so high that the compression of air developed by injection is not sufficient to push the air into the esophagus. If inhalation is tried, the PE segment may not be relaxed sufficiently to permit atmospheric air pressure to insufflate the esophagus. Dilation of the PE stricture has been tried with some success in achieving esophageal sound production (Damsté, 1979). There appears to be a relation between PE relaxation for deglutition and air intake. Volin (1980) reported that postoperative difficulty in swallowing due to PE stricture was a significant predictor of esophageal speech failure.

As discussed previously, the striated PE segment is under both reflexive and voluntary control of the central nervous system, but the exact nature of this control is not well understood. Based on his electromyographic (EMG) studies of the inferior constrictor and cricopharyngeus muscles, Shipp (1970) suggested that poor esophageal speakers had less voluntary control over the "velocity and magnitude of pharyngoesophageal muscle contraction" (p. 192) than did adequate speakers. How esophageal speakers acquire this voluntary control over the PE segment for phonation purposes is unknown.

Extraneous Noises

In addition to working on rapid and smooth air intake, the patient should try to eliminate extraneous noises that may accompany the insufflation or exsufflation of esophageal air. The two major extraneous noises are klunking, which may occur in those individuals who use the injection process, and a high-pitched rushing noise, usually heard in inhalers.

As air is pumped by the tongue down into the hypopharynx, through the PE segment, and into the esophagus, a "klunk" may be perceived immediately before the attempt at phonation. The klunk seems to be exaggerated when the injection is done under tension. However, klunking also has been observed to persist long after the patient has become proficient and relaxed during injected air intake.

How and when klunking occurs are important. Diedrich and Youngstrom (1966) indicated that when the tongue retrudes, it frequently occludes the hypopharynx; they speculated that when the tongue moves forward, it may leave a partial vacuum. As air rushes in to fill this void, a klunking sound may be produced. Sometimes when the hypopharynx is not occluded, a klunk is still heard; consequently, the sound also may be produced when air fills the esophagus.

Evidence for the latter statement comes from Shipp (1970). Electrodes were connected to the inferior constrictor and the cricopharyngeus muscle during surgery. About 1 month after surgery, EMG tracings were made during air intake. The injection method of esophageal inflation was signaled by a klunk. Firing of the inferior constrictor and/or cricopharyngeus muscles was usually noted during injection of air. The recorded EMG activity was interpreted by Shipp as either brief stretch reflexes or active contractions of these muscles to propel the bolus of air into the esophagus. In either case, the reason for the klunk—air expansion or compression of the hypopharyngeal (inferior constrictor) and/or the cricopharyngeal musculature—is unclear. Another interesting observation was that klunking was heard on initial air intake before a phrase, or during an interphrase pause, but was not heard on consonant injection of air intake that occurred during the utterance of an intraphrase interval. If a laryngectomized patient is asked to produce a series of pa-pa-pa syllables, a klunk may be heard before the first pa, but rarely on successive pa utterances.

To summarize, klunking usually is heard with injection but not inhalation; klunking may be the result of air filling a partial vacuum in the cavity of either the hypopharynx or the esophagus; and klunking generally occurs when air is injected at the beginning of a phrase, but not with consonant press injection during a phrase. These observations illustrate differences in the physiology of air intake phenomena.

Management tactics that are sometimes successful in eliminating the klunk are to encourage a relaxed air intake mode or to make the patient aware of the initial injection of air and contrast it with the multiple air intakes of the pa-pa-pa syllables. The goal is for the patient to distinguish differences in the tongue and/or throat movements and mimic those movements that do not elicit a klunk during air intake. Knox, Eccleston, Maurer, and Gordon (1987) determined that intake noise (klunk) acceptability was not a significant correlate of overall esophageal speech proficiency. They recommended that clinicians concentrate on other speech parameters, such as duration (increase syllables per injection), quality, and inflection.

The other major extraneous noise—the high-pitched rushing sound—occurs through the stoma. The sound is associated primarily with pulmonary exhalation, although in some individuals it may also be heard in pulmonary inspiration. Also, stoma noises are more commonly associated with inhalers than with injectors. When esophageal phonation takes place, the respiratory exhalation usually is synchronized with the effort at esophageal phonation. The high-pitched rushing noise (turbulence) is heard as the exhaled air is forced out of the narrow stoma. A similar noise is heard when the patient attempts to clear any mucus that may have accumulated in the trachea. The clinician's first step in eliminating this sound is to make the patient aware of the sound by means of auditory discrimination. Next, the clinician asks the patient to produce esophageal sound with less pulmonary effort. Also, the clinician encourages attempts to increase the duration of the esophageal sound and to use less intensity (loudness), rather than to make a quick, sharp burst of esophageal sound. Sometimes the patient can find it useful to attend to a slow squeeze rather than a quick contraction of the abdominal muscles. The patient can feel his or her own abdominal muscles while practicing quick–slow pulmonary exhalation alone. Next, the clinician has the patient add attempts at achieving esophageal tone with slow pulmonary exhalation.

Some laryngectomees who learn to inhale air into the esophagus may produce an esophageal-like tone as the air passes from the vocal tract through the PE segment into the esophagus. A comparable analogy exists in laryngeal individuals when inspiratory noises (stridor) are produced by the larynx during inhalation. When laryngectomees are made aware of this sound, most seem capable of readjusting the manner of air intake so that the PE segment no longer vibrates on inhalation.

A watery (gurgly) esophageal sound is generally due to excessive mucus on the superior surface of the PE segment. Patients report that the consistency of the mucus appears to be thickened by milk or milk products, making the mucus more difficult to swallow. Drinking hot black coffee or tea or sucking a hard candy seems to make the mucus easier to swallow.

A loss in auditory sensitivity may preclude the patient from hearing any of the above extraneous noises. Poor speech has been found to be related to the severity of the sensory neural loss (Diedrich & Youngstrom, 1966, pp. 54ff). Consequently, an audiometric assessment is an indispensable evaluative tool.

Speed of Air Intake

One objective in esophageal speech training is to have less than a 1-s latency between the beginning of the air intake attempt and the production of esophageal sound (Berlin, 1963, 1965). Damsté (1958) reported air intake to average 0.21 s in 23 patients. Diedrich and Youngstrom (1966) found air intake speed to be approximately 0.50 s, and another 0.20 s (prephonation time) occurred before speech was heard. The clinician should encourage smooth air intake. The patient should avoid uncoordinated movements, start–stop actions of the tongue or jaw, and asynchrony with respiration in the air intake maneuver. To the listener, the proficient speaker demonstrates minimal overt motor activity of the peripheral oral structures. This activity takes considerable practice and may take many months to master.

Another goal for esophageal speakers is to maximize the duration of phonation. Berlin (1965) reported that good speakers sustained the vowel /a/ for an average of 2.37 s whereas poor speakers averaged 0.98 s. This may not seem like much considering normal speakers may sustain /a/ for more than 15 s. However, Jaffe and Feldstein (1970, p. 22) noted that, in normal speech interchange, the "rhythmical unit in talking is a string of 2–10 words, averaging 5," with a mean duration of approximately 1.64 s in natural dialogue. Hesitation and juncture pauses ranged from .66 to .77 s. Esophageal speakers spoke at approximately 2 words/second, compared with 2.5 words/second for normal speakers (Snidecor & Isshiki, 1965a). Accounting for somewhat slower articulation rates, 4-word utterances are possible in 2 s for the esophageal speaker.

As noted earlier, the esophagus has a limited capacity ranging from 40 to 80 cc. Up to 50 cc of air may enter and leave the esophagus (Isshiki & Snidecor, 1965). In their study of belching in normal speakers, Kahrilas et al. (1986) instilled 30 ml of air into the esophagus and found that a belch occurred 0.5 s after the air distended the esophagus. The belch lasted for 1.4 s. A swallow-induced relaxation of the PE segment lasted less than 0.3 s, and a belch-related relaxation lasted 1.2 s. Kahrilas et al. observed an almost linear function between the volume (5, 10, 15, and 30 ml) of air injected into the esophagus and the duration of relaxation in the PE segment pressure zone. In other words, the larger the volume, the longer the PE pressure zone remained relaxed.

In a study of retrospective and prospective postlaryngectomized patients who learned esophageal speech, Ryan, Gates, Cantu, and Hearne (1982) collected measures on the maximum sustained duration of phonation of /a/ and syllables/second from a single injection of air into the esophagus. For 22 esophageal speaking subjects who were studied retrospectively (more than 6 years after their laryngectomies), the mean phonation duration was 2.11 s (SD ± 0.64). These subjects produced 7.1 syllables (SD ± 0.64) per air injection. In the 12 laryngectomized subjects who developed esophageal speech in the 6 months after completion of their cancer therapy, mean phonation duration was 1.16 s (SD ± 0.15) and mean syllables per injection was 6.0 (SD ± 1.1). Therefore, despite the limited air supply and unique neoglottis, esophageal speakers who can sustain phonation for approximately 2 s can utter phrases that appear to be within normal expectations.

OTHER SPEECH-RELATED ISSUES

Articulatory Performance

It once was thought that the laryngectomee needed only to acquire an alternate voice and then articulate in the "usual" manner to produce esophageal speech. However, the gestures necessary for articulation have been modified. Studies of vowel duration (Christiansen & Weinberg, 1976), oral pressures (Swisher, 1980), voice onset time (VOT) (Christiansen, Weinberg, & Alfonso, 1978), and initiation and termination of voicing (Sacco, Mann, & Schultz, 1967) all indicated differences between laryngeal speakers and esophageal speakers in producing phonological contrasts.

Voiceless Sounds. The production of voiceless plosives and sibilants are particularly affected in esophageal speech. The /p/ sound is made by approximating the lips, establishing velopharyngeal closure, and building up intraoral air pressure in the vocal tract with air exhaled from the lungs. How can laryngectomees do this? They cannot, because air is no longer available via the pulmonary system (lungs) since the trachea is diverted from the hypopharynx and sewn to the base of the neck (Figure 1.1). For the laryngectomee to produce the /p/, air pressure must be developed within the oral cavity and released past the lips. Try producing the /p/ sound with your lips closed and without using air from your lungs. An aspirate /p/ can be produced with intraoral air pressure. Although similar, the sound produced is not perceptually the same as the pulmonary-produced aspirate /p/. Make these voiceless sounds /t,k,f,s, ʃ,tʃ/ in both the intraoral and pulmonary manner. In conversational speech with a laryngectomee, the listener makes the necessary perceptual adjustments and has little difficulty understanding the esophageal speech produced.

Voiced Sounds. When the /b/ sound is made, the laryngectomee must coordinate the PE vibration with the necessary intraoral air pressure to make the sound distinguishable. Swisher (1980) studied oral pressures in both laryngeal and esophageal speakers. The oral pressures for the voiceless /p/ (7.0 cm/H$_2$0) were greater than the voiced /b/ (3.5 cm/H$_2$0) in laryngeal speakers. Not only did esophageal speakers have much higher pressures for /p/ (35.6 cm/H$_2$0) and /b/ (33.4 cm/H$_2$0), but the voiced pressures were nearly as high as the voiceless. In addition, Christiansen et al. (1978) clearly demonstrated shorter VOT lag intervals in esophageal than in normal speakers for all the prevocalic voiceless /p,t,k/ stop comparisons, but no differences were found between the two groups for the voiced /b,d,g/ comparisons.

Nasal Sounds. Several studies have demonstrated that the nasal sounds in esophageal speech are perceived as denasal (b/m,d/n). In cinefluorographic studies, Diedrich and Youngstrom (1966) discovered that most of the esophageal speakers kept their velopharyngeal (v-p) mechanism consistently closed during speech, which explains why nasals are perceived as denasal. The speakers may have adapted this strategy because most esophageal speakers use the injection technique for trapping/pushing air into the esophagus. Recall that during injection the v-p mechanism must be closed in order for the compressed air to be directed into the hypopharynx and then to the esophagus. Otherwise, the compressed air would escape into the nasal cavities. The esophageal speaker subconsciously decides, "I'll keep my v-p mechanism closed throughout all speech attempts." Similarly, the young child learns to open and close the v-p mechanism quite unconsciously while developing the nasal sounds.

Recently, Miller and Hamlet (1988), in a study on nasal consonants in esophageal speech, found that amount of nasal resonance was a function of word position and time following injection of esophageal air. Nasal resonance measured with a nasal accelerometer was higher on nasal consonants in word-final position (e.g., *assume*) than in word-initial position (e.g., *movie*). The authors suggested that most esophageal speakers curtail velopharyngeal openness on nasal consonants. If the nasal consonant were in the initial position or used in the injection of air, then complete denasalization might occur.

Vowels. In addition to changes made by esophageal speakers in the articulation of consonants, vowels are modified. Swisher (1980) reported that the mean phonation time for vowels in esophageal speakers was increased, sometimes more than twice as long as in laryngeal speakers. Esophageal speakers whose vowel durations were shorter (or more like the laryngeal speakers) were judged more intelligible.

Sisty and Weinberg (1972) observed higher vowel formant frequency characteristics in male and female esophageal speakers than in normal speakers. These investigators suggested that removal of the larynx may shorten the vocal tract. They cited Diedrich and Youngstrom (1966), who found in a patient studied 20 months postoperatively that the hypopharynx was shorter during esophageal phonation than it had been during preoperative laryngeal phonation.

Pitch and Loudness of Esophageal Phonation

Mean fundamental frequency ranges of 50 to 100 Hz (Van den Berg & Moolenaar-Bijl, 1959) and 29 to 37 Hz (Perry & Tikofsky, 1965) have been reported in esophageal speakers. Curry and Snidecor (1961) found a median fundamental frequency of 63 Hz (range 17–135 Hz). Shipp's (1967) better speakers had a mean of 84.4 Hz, whereas poorer speakers had a mean of 64.7 Hz. Some unusual esophageal speakers are capable of producing an octave range of pitch variation. Most are capable of some upward and downward variation in stress and inflection. Van den Berg and Moolenaar-Bijl (1959) believed that the good speaker can give the illusion of changes in pitch by modifying the vocal cavities in such a way that the resonant frequencies (formants) are changed during the production of a vowel.

Hyman (1955) measured loudness (intensity) and found normal speakers at 29 dB and esophageal speakers at 23 dB using a reference level of 50 dB re 0.0002 dynes/cm². McKinley (1960) reported that the average intensity of esophageal speech was about 6 to 7 dB below that of normal speech. Van den Berg and Moolenaar-Bijl (1959) reported that pitch and intensity were correlated in esophageal speech: low pitch with low intensity and high pitch with high intensity (increased flow of air through the pseudoglottis). Snidecor and Isshiki (1965b) assumed that the mean flow rate in esophageal speakers was more important for intensity than in normal speakers. If their conclusions are correct, loudness of esophageal speech is dependent upon the expulsion rate and the amount of air that is capable of being trapped in the esophagus. To obtain increased intensity at a high pitch, the flow rate must be increased. Since esophageal speakers have only one-third the flow rate of normal speakers, it is little wonder that they frequently do not obtain good intensity levels at higher pitches. Knox et al. (1987) reported that intensity of esophageal speech was not highly correlated with esophageal speech proficiency. They suggested that consideration should be made of other speech intelligibility variables, such as rate and duration of phonation (syllables/air charge).

All of these studies suggest that a laryngectomy affects not only the source of sound, pitch, and loudness, but also other speech functions (resonance, consonants, and vowels).

PRODUCING MULTIPLE SYLLABLES

Two important physiological determinants for producing multiple syllables are the amount of air supply insufflated into the esophagus and the manner(s) of air intake.

Capacity of the Esophagus

The capacity of the esophagus has been estimated to range from 40 to 80 cc. Isshiki and Snidecor (1965) demonstrated that up to 50 cc of air may enter the esophagus during one air trap maneuver, and the same amount usually leaves the esophagus during phonation. Ryan et al. (1982) found that esophageal speakers averaged six to seven syllables per injection. Obviously, if patients are limited in the amount of air that they can insufflate into the esophagus, then their duration of phonation also is limited. If the phonation is less than 1 s, few multiple syllables are possible.

Manner of Air Intake

In the beginning of esophageal speech training, patients (may) learn how to inhale and/or inject air into the esophagus before producing a /pa/ or an /a/ sound. After learning how to do this, some patients learn (on their own or with instruction) how to inject air from certain consonants into the esophagus. Studies have demonstrated that when patients produce sounds that require high intraoral air pressure (e.g., especially the voiceless /p,t,k,s/), some of the impounded air in the vocal tract may be injected into the esophagus (Diedrich & Youngstrom, 1966; Van den Berg et al., 1958). This maneuver has been described as a consonant press. Consequently, it is possible to make a string of /pa-pa-pa . . . pa/ syllables whereby, immediately preceding each /p/ sound, some air is injected into the esophagus and used for the phonation of the vowel /a/. The laryngectomee who does this can take a respiratory (pulmonary) breath and produce repetitive pa-pa sounds until all of the pulmonary air is consumed (expired). This pulmonary exhalation may last 10–15 s, while simultaneously producing multiple consonant–vowel units. Moolenaar-Bijl (1953) found that 1 subject could produce as many as 20 to 40 /p,t, or k/ sounds in one intake of air, but only 7 to 8 /m,l,b, or d/ sounds. Berlin (1965) reported that esophageal speakers could produce multiple /da/ sounds about 1 s longer than the /a/ sound (the mean time increased from 2.49 to 3.69 s). Diedrich and Youngstrom (1966) observed that it is possible to produce the frication sound for /s/ and to simultaneously inject air into the esophagus.

Some patients inhale air into the esophagus preceding the word and make use of the consonant press within the word. For example, they may say the word *carpenter,* (inhale) *car* – (consonant press) *pen* – (consonant press) *ter.* Other patients may inject air before the word (without the consonant) and then use a consonant press within the word: (inject) *car* – (consonant press) *pen* – (consonant press) *ter.* The blends (/sp/, /st/, /sk/) and affricate /tʃ/ also seem useful in consonant air injection. It appears to be more difficult to inject air when a voiced plosive–sibilant is used than when a voiceless plosive–sibilant is used. Air injection from plosive–sibilant sounds is usually noted in the initial (releasing) position rather than in the final (arresting) position of a syllable pulse. Use of the consonant press within a word or phrase enables the esophageal speaker to lengthen phrases, thus appearing more normal in speech output.

Diedrich and Youngstrom's (1966, pp. 94ff) study of cinefluorograms revealed interesting patterns of movement for the tongue tip, posterior tongue, palate, and PE segment. The similarity of the air intake maneuver from a posture of rest and during an *interphrase* pause was striking (Figure 1.4A, B, and C). Furthermore, during the continuous utterance, no tongue tip alveolar contact was noted during the *intraphrase* consonant-press insufflation (Figure 1.4D). The distance between the posterior tongue and the pharyngeal wall also was consistently shorter for air intake during the intraphrase utterance; and the PE segment was consistently placed in a caudal direction (D). These observations illuminated the differences in morphology and the amazing adaptive physiology that occurs after laryngectomy to permit air intake in esophageal speech.

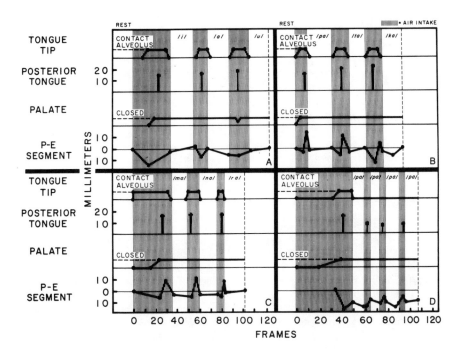

Figure 1.4. Vocal tract movements. These graphs illustrate the movement patterns of tongue tip to alveolar ridge, posterior tongue to posterior pharyngeal wall, velopharyngeal closure, and cephalad and caudad movement of the superior surface of the pharyngo-esophageal (P-E) segment from a position of rest. The amount of movement is expressed in millimeters and the temporal rate is 24 frames per second. L22 is depicted phonating four sequences: (A) /i/, /a/, /u/; (B) /pa/, /ta/, /ka/; (C) /ma/, /na/, /ra/; and (D) a series of /papapapa/ sounds. In Sequences A, B, and C, L22 had an interphrase pause for air intake before each phonation. During Sequence D, he had no overt characteristics of air intake yet was replenishing his esophageal air supply during the intraphrase pauses.

Sequences A, B, and C illustrate the similarity of the morphological dynamics when air intake takes place from a posture of rest and when air intake occurs during the interphrase pause. Sequence D illustrates the differences in air intake which takes place from rest and air intake which occurs during the intraphrase interval. During the latter, the tongue tip is not used, the posterior tongue is closer to the pharyngeal wall, and the P-E segment is consistently displaced in a caudal direction.

The palate is closed from the first air intake until the end of the phonations. Even on the nasal consonants, no break in velopharyngeal closure is noted. For clarity in the diagram and to emphasize the differences noted in the two air intakes, the movements of the tongue are indicated only during air intake and not during phonation. From *Alaryngeal Speech* (p. 101) by W. M. Diedrich and K. A. Youngstrom, 1966, Springfield, IL: Charles C. Thomas. Reprinted by permission.

ACKNOWLEDGMENT

The author acknowledges with gratitude those students and staff who read and provided helpful suggestions to improve the clarity of this manuscript. Any unclear statements that remain are my responsibility.

REFERENCES

Atkinson, M., Kramer, P., Wyman, S. M., & Inglefinger, F. J. (1957). The dynamics of swallowing: I. Normal pharyngeal mechanisms. *Journal of Clinical Investigation, 36,* 581–588.

Berlin, C. I. (1963). Clinical measurement of esophageal speech: I. Methodology and curves of skill acquisition. *Journal of Speech and Hearing Disorders, 28,* 42–51.

Berlin, C. I. (1965). Clinical measurement of esophageal speech: III. Performance of nonbiased groups. *Journal of Speech and Hearing Disorders, 30,* 174–183.

Bosone-Crouch, Z. (1974). *The relationship of intraluminal swallowing, resting, and phonation pressures, to esophageal phonation "goodness" and maximum duration of phonation.* Unpublished doctoral dissertation, University of Kansas, Lawrence.

Christiansen, J. M., & Weinberg, B. (1976). Vowel duration characteristics of esophageal speech. *Journal of Speech and Hearing Research, 19,* 678–689.

Christiansen, J. M., Weinberg, B., & Alfonso, P. J. (1978). Productive voice onset time characteristics of esophageal speech. *Journal of Speech and Hearing Research, 21,* 56–72.

Curry, E. T., & Snidecor, J. C. (1961). Physical measurement and pitch perception in esophageal speech. *Laryngoscope, 71,* 415–424.

Damsté, P. H. (1958). *Oesophageal speech after laryngectomy.* Groningen, The Netherlands: Gebroeders Hoitsema.

Damsté, P. H. (1979). Some obstacles in learning esophageal speech. In R. L. Keith & F. L. Darley (Eds.), *Laryngectomee rehabilitation.* Austin, TX: PRO-ED.

Damsté, P. H., Van den Berg, J., & Moolenaar-Bijl, A. J. (1956). Why are some patients unable to learn esophageal speech? *Annals of Otology, Rhinology and Laryngology, 65,* 998–1005.

Decroix, G., Libersa, C., & Lattard, R. (1958). Bases anatomiques et physiologiques de la reeducation vocale des laryngectomisés [The anatomical and physiological foundations of voice reeducation in laryngectomees]. *Journal of Francais d'Otorhinolaryngologie, 7,* 549–573.

Dey, F. L., & Kirchner, J. A. (1961). The upper esophageal sphincter after laryngectomy. *Laryngoscope, 71,* 99–115.

Diedrich, W. M. (1968). The mechanism of esophageal speech. *Annals of the New York Academy of Sciences, 155,* 303–317.

Diedrich, W. M., & Youngstrom, K. A. (1966). *Alaryngeal speech.* Springfield, IL: Charles C. Thomas.

Ekberg, O. (1986). The cricopharyngeus revisited. *The British Journal of Radiology, 59,* 875–879.

Gates, G. A. (1980). Upper esophageal sphincter: Pre- and post-laryngectomy— A normative study. *Laryngoscope, 90,* 454–464.

Gates, G. A., Ryan, W., Cantu, E., & Hearne, E. (1982). Current status of laryngectomee rehabilitation: II. Causes of failure. *American Journal of Otolaryngology, 3,* 8–14.

Gerhardt, D., Hewett, J., Moeschberger, M., Shuck, T., & Winship, D. (1980). Human upper esophageal sphincter pressure profile. *American Journal of Physiology, 239,* G49–G52.

Hixon, T. J. (1973). Respiratory function in speech. In F. Minifie, T. J. Nixon, & F. Williams (Eds.), *Normal aspects of speech, hearing, and language* (pp. 73–125). Englewood Cliffs, NJ: Prentice-Hall.

Hyman, M. (1955). An experimental study of artificial larynx and esophageal speech. *Journal of Speech and Hearing Disorders, 20,* 291–299.

Inglefinger, F. J. (1958). Esophageal motility. *Physiology Review, 38,* 533–584.

Isshiki, N., & Snidecor, J. C. (1965). Air intake and usage in esophageal speech. *Acta Otolaryngology, 59,* 559–574.

Jaffe, J., & Feldstein, S. (1970). *Rhythms of dialogue.* New York: Academic Press.

Kahrilas, P. J., Dodds, W. J., Dent, J., Wyman, J. B., Hogan, W. J., & Arndoffer, R. C. (1986). Upper esophageal sphincter function during belching. *Gastroenterology, 91,* 133–140.

Knox, A. W., Eccleston, V., Maurer, J. F., & Gordon, M. C. (1987). Correlates of sophisticated listener judgments of esophageal air intake noise. *Journal of Communication Disorders, 20,* 25–39.

Kramer, P., Atkinson, M., Syman, S. M., & Inglefinger, J. J. (1957). The dynamics of swallowing: II. Neuromuscular dysphagia of the pharynx. *Journal of Clinical Investigation, 36,* 589–595.

Loudon, R. G., Lee, L., & Holcomb, B. J. (1988). Volumes and breathing patterns during speech in healthy and asthmatic subjects. *Journal of Speech and Hearing Research, 31,* 219–227.

McKinley, S. (1960). *Correlates of stress patterns in esophageal speech.* Unpublished master's thesis, Vanderbilt University, Nashville, TN.

Miller, W. L., & Hamlet, S. L. (1988). Nasal consonants in esophageal speech. *Journal of Speech and Hearing Disorders, 53,* 108–111.

Moolenaar-Bijl, A. J. (1953). Connection between consonant articulation and the intake of air in esophageal speech. *Folia Phoniatrica, 5,* 212–215.

Payne, W. S., & Olsen, A. M. (1974). *The esophagus.* Philadelphia: Lea & Febiger.

Perry, P. S., & Tikofsky, R. S. (1965). The occurrence of low valued, weak intensity frequencies in normal and esophageal phonation. In R. S. Tikofsky (Ed.), *Phonetic characteristics of esophageal speech* (Appendix VI) (ORA Project No. 05539). Ann Arbor, MI: University of Michigan, Office of Research Administration.

Ryan, W., Gates, G. A., Cantu, E., & Hearne, E. M. (1982). Current status of laryngectomee rehabilitation: III. Understanding of esophageal speech. *American Journal of Otolaryngology, 3,* 91–96.

Sacco, P. R., Mann, M. B., & Schultz, M. C. (1967). Perceptual confusions among selected phonemes in esophageal speech. *Journal of the Indiana Speech and Hearing Association, 26,* 19–33.

Shipp, T. (1967). Frequency, duration, and perceptual measures in relation to judgments of alaryngeal speech acceptability. *Journal of Speech and Hearing Research, 10,* 417–427.

Shipp, T. (1970). EMG of pharyngoesophageal musculature during alaryngeal voice production. *Journal of Speech Hearing Research, 13,* 184–192.

Sisty, N. L., & Weinberg, B. (1972). Formant frequency characteristics of esophageal speech. *Journal of Speech and Hearing Research, 15,* 439–448.

Snidecor, J. C., & Isshiki, N. (1965a). Air volume and air flow relationships of six male esophageal speakers. *Journal of Speech and Hearing Disorders, 30,* 205–216.

Snidecor, J. C., & Isshiki, N. (1965b). Vocal and air use characteristics of a superior male esophageal speaker. *Folia Phoniatrica, 17,* 217–232.

Snidecor, J. C., and Others. (1969). *Speech rehabilitation of the laryngectomized* (2nd ed.). Springfield, IL: Charles C. Thomas.

Storchi, O. F., & Micheli-Pellegrini, V. (1959). A proposito dell'innervazione ricorrenziale del muscolo cricofaringeo e della sua importanza nella fonazione dei laringectomizzati. *Bollettino delle malattie dell'oreccho, della golla, del naso, 77,* 3–14.

Swisher, W. E. (1980). Oral pressures, vowel durations, and acceptability ratings of esophageal speakers. *Journal of Communication Disorders, 13,* 171–181.

Van den Berg, J., & Moolenaar-Bijl, A. J. (1959). Cricopharyngeal sphincter, pitch, intensity, and fluency in oesophageal speech. *Practica Oto-rhino-laryngologica, 21,* 298–315.

Van den Berg, J., Moolenaar-Bijl, A. J., & Damsté, P. H. (1958). Oesophageal speech. *Folia Phoniatrica, 10,* 65–84.

Volin, R. A. (1980). Predicting failure to speak after laryngectomy. *Laryngoscope, 90,* 1727–1736.

Welch, R. W., Gates, G. A., Luckmann, K. F., Ricks, P. M., & Drake, S. T. (1979). Change in the force-summed pressure measurements of the upper esophageal sphincter prelaryngectomy and postlaryngectomy. *Annals of Otolaryngology, 88,* 804–808.

Welch, R. W., Luckmann, K., Ricks, P. M., Drake, S. T., & Gates, G. A. (1979). Manometry of the upper esophageal sphincter and its alterations in laryngectomy. *Journal of Clinical Investigation, 63,* 1036–1041.

Winans, C. S., Reichbach, E. J., & Waldrop, W. F. (1974). Esophageal determinants of alaryngeal speech. *Archives of Otolaryngology, 99,* 10–14.

Zaino, C., Jacobson, H. G., Lepow, H., & Ozturk, C. H. (1970). *The pharyngoesophageal sphincter.* Springfield, IL: Charles C. Thomas.

CHAPTER 2

The Artificial Larynx

Jay W. Lerman

> *Lerman stresses the value of early introduction to artificial larynx devices. He discusses the stages of therapy from initial sound production to refinement and provides a valuable guide to troubleshooting malfunction of the speech aids.*

Study Questions

1. *What is the rationale for using an artificial larynx?*
2. *What types of artificial larynges are available?*
3. *What parameters of speech contribute most to intelligibility with the artificial larynx and why?*

This chapter describes the artificial larynx devices and explains how they are used in the rehabilitation of the laryngectomized patient. The intention is not to answer all of the questions that may occur during the teaching of artificial larynx speech, but rather to present a personal clinical point of view and a base from which each clinician may begin to function.

The material presented is based primarily on patient needs as perceived during my clinical experience. Although some aspects of the management process may be controversial in relation to present treatment philosophy, this discussion is intended to introduce the clinician to some of the basic principles of management with an artificial larynx.

A detailed description of the anatomy and physiology associated with laryngectomy was presented in chapter 1. The following information is presented very simply to facilitate understanding of the relationship of the larynx to phonation and its other functions.

It must be remembered that the larynx has functions more vital than phonation. Its primary role is to act as a sphincter to protect the airway and to take part in respiration. When an individual is laryngectomized, respiration no longer occurs through the larynx. As a patient once reported, "My nose is on my neck." Certainly, the function of phonation, as we normally perceive it, also changes radically following a laryngectomy, as the patient is left with no voice. Phonation can be accomplished without a larynx, however, through esophageal speech, speech resulting from tracheoesophageal fistulization, and artificial larynx speech. This chapter is concerned with speech rehabilitation through the use of an artificial larynx.

HISTORICAL REVIEW

Although most writings have credited Gussenbauer (1874) with creating the first artificial larynx for a laryngectomee, Czermak (1859) reported on an artificial larynx provided to a tracheotomized woman in 1859. The early artificial larynges used pulmonary air, usually exhaled from the tracheostoma to a tube containing a vibrating reed. The laryngectomee articulated the artificial sound that was introduced into the mouth. Over the years, improvements have been made on the instrumentation. With the advent of the electronic larynx, the reed type of artificial larynx fell into disuse. However, in the past 15 years, with the establishment of the Tokyo artificial larynx and others, a resurgence has occurred in the use of this reed-type instrument. (For a more complete history of the artificial larynx, see Blom, 1979; Lebrun, 1973; Lowry, 1981.) According to Lebrun (1973),

The first electrolarynx seems to have been devised by Gluck. In 1909 [he] showed the members of the Laryngological Society in Berlin an electric prosthesis comprising a phonograph of the Edison type driven by an electro-motor and connected with a receiver that was fitted into the patient's nose or attached to his denture. On the cylinder of the phonograph a vowel, i.e., a succession of damped oscillations, produced by a singer had been recorded. When the recording was played back, each damped oscillation in the record originated an electric current that energized the membrane of the receiver. The movements to and fro of the membrane caused the air in the buccal cavity to vibrate. (pp. 56–57)

Not until the 1940s was a viable and usable electrolarynx introduced (Greene, 1942a, 1942b). Since that time, a wide variety of electrolarynges have been developed (Blom, 1978).

TYPES OF ARTIFICIAL LARYNGES

Artificial larynges generally have been divided into two types, pneumatic and electronic. The electrolarynx has been subdivided further into intraoral (mouth-type) and transcervical (neck-type). To appreciate better the value of the artificial larynx, the clinician should try to "obtain first hand experience with each of the instruments" and to "become proficient at using them" (Blom, 1978).

Pneumatic Larynges

With the pneumatic artificial larynx, pulmonary air travels up through the tracheostoma and into the voice prosthesis, which has been placed over the patient's stoma. The pulmonary air sets a reed or other membrane into vibration, producing a tone that is delivered directly into the patient's mouth via an intraoral tube. The patient can then articulate this tone.

Several pneumatic artificial larynges have been available, including the Japanese-made Tokyo and Osaka models, and the Van Humen DSP8 from the Netherlands. The Japanese devices, which cost about $49 each, come with additional mouth tube, air tube, NEW Welch stoma cushion, two sheets of diaphragm rubber, and a 60-min training tape. They can be purchased from Clyde Welch, 2027 Read Street #53, Omaha, NE 68112. The DSP8, rarely seen in the United States, is available for about $85 from Memacon, Pres. Kennedylaan 263, P.O. Box 56, Velp 6200, Netherlands.

Electrolarynges

Intraoral Type (Mouth-Type). The battery-operated intraoral instrument transmits an electronically generated tone to the mouth of the patient, via a mouth tube. The speaker then modifies the tone through articulation into speech. The most popular intraoral instrument has been the Cooper-Rand Electronic Speech Aid, which can be obtained for about $295 from Luminaud, 8688 Tyler Boulevard, Mentor, OH 44060.

Recently, however, another intraoral electrolarynx has been developed and marketed. The Companion—much smaller, lighter, and less expensive than the Cooper-Rand—can be obtained for about $130 from E.Z. Speech Inc., P.O. Box 1758, Richmond, VA 23214.

In addition, manufacturers of the Servox and Aurex neck-type instruments have made adaptation kits that allow for conversion from transcervical into intraoral devices. These conversion kits add between $10 and $20 to the basic cost of the instrument.

Transcervical Type (Neck-Type). The electronic neck-type instrument is the most commonly used artificial larynx in the United States. The most popular model is the Western Electric #5 (Salmon & Goldstein, 1978). Neck-type artificial larynges are hand held, are battery operated, and have an electronically activated sound source. When the vibrating source is correctly placed against the neck, sound is transmitted into the vocal tract. The patient then modifies this tone through articulation in a manner similar to that with an intraoral device.

Although many neck-type artificial larynges are available, the four most widely used in this country are the Western Electric #5C, available for about $130 by calling the AT&T Special Needs Center in New Jersey at (800) 233-1222; the Servox Inton, which can be obtained for about $559 from the Siemens Corporation, 10 Constitution Avenue, Piscapaway, NJ 08855; the Aurex Neovox, which is available for about $405 from the Aurex Corporation, 315 South Peoria Street, Chicago, IL 60607; and the ROMET, which is available from either Laryngectomy Supply Co., 461 SW 156th Street, Seattle, WA 98166, or ROMET, Inc., Hawaii Kai Corporate Plaza, #221, 6600 Kalanianaole Highway, Honolulu, HI 96825. The approximate cost for the ROMET is $395 and includes two rechargeable batteries and a charger.

In recent years, both Western Electric and Servox have modified their instruments. Western Electric has altered their device so that a 9-V battery can be used instead of two 5.6-V batteries, reducing operating cost. However, in making this modification, they eliminated the external variable pitch control so that through an internal adjustment only one preset pitch is available to users.

DR. Kuhn & Co. recently developed the Servox Inton. The older, standard Servox model had pitch and volume controls. The Servox Inton has a volume control and two control buttons for production of two pitches. An internal adjustment of the basic pitch of the upper button automatically adjusts the pitch produced by the lower button; the lower button produces a sound one-half tone higher in pitch than that of the top button. The manufacturer points out that with proper use, a minimal number of prosodic features are available for questions, rhythm, and melody. In addition, the instrument can be adjusted for a continuous decrease in pitch, which occurs automatically when the lower of the control buttons is depressed. The manufacturer suggests that this "automatic tone decay" together with the secondary pitch allows for more normal sounding speech.

To set the fundamental frequency for the top button, remove the battery cover and the battery. Then, place the battery holder on a flat surface and press down on the outer case until it begins to slide off. Remove this case to expose the internal mechanism. Leaving the outer case off, replace the battery and battery cover. The fundamental pitch adjustment screw can be turned only with the Teflon™ screwdriver provided, until the preferred pitch is determined.

For additional adjustment of the automatic tone decay, the grey plastic panel covering the circuit board must be lifted off, the Phillips™ screw is removed and the edge of the panel near the screw is lifted carefully, allowing the panel to slide outward. Care must be taken to prevent damage to the mechanism. All adjustment screws are labeled. Complete instructions may be obtained from the manufacturer, DR. Kuhn & Co., Munich, or the U.S. distributing agent, Siemens Hearing Instruments, Inc., Piscapaway, NJ.

Lowry (1981) reported on a self-contained intraoral artificial larynx called Speechmaster Intraoral Artificial Larynx. This instrument was designed to be contained within the oral cavity with a dental prosthesis. For a variety of reasons (cost, loudness, hygiene, etc.), manufacture of this instrument has been abandoned.

This attempt by Lowry to introduce a different type of speech aid raises an interesting issue. Except for the Servox Inton and the Speechmaster Intraoral devices, no unique models have been developed since 1959. Technical issues mentioned in the 1950s (Barney, 1958; Barney, Haworth, & Dunn, 1959)—such as acoustic factors that influence speech quality, consonant production, and speech understandability—have not been fully addressed by manufacturers. Weinberg (1981) also discussed several attributes for manufacturers to incorporate into artificial laryngeal devices: inconspicuousness, dependability, reasonable cost, simplicity of operation, hygienic acceptability, as well as capability for achieving quality, prosody, and intensity comparable to that of normal speech.

Obviously, no available electronic device meets *all* the specified requirements or desirable attributes. The ROMET is smaller, lighter

in weight, and somewhat less conspicuous than the others. Newly introduced saliva filters and cord guards have improved the Cooper-Rand
so this intraoral device now requires fewer repairs. Battery chargers
for all neck-type devices except the Western Electric #5C and the change
to a more commonly used voltage reduce cost. With other modifications,
some devices are simpler to operate, except for the new Servox Inton.

Despite the advent of digitizing and microcomputer chip technology,
improved quality and intonation features of artificial larynges have not
been addressed. As Weinberg (1981) so aptly stated,

> An unfortunate commentary would unfold if, over the next decade, society
> came to accept and gracefully interact with a multitude of devices that 'speak'
> using artificially generated stimuli, while at the same time, laryngectomized
> people, with intact articulatory and linguistic competence, continued to
> produce speech using methods that are not this acceptable. (p. 146)

CANDIDACY

The question is not who is a suitable candidate for an artificial larynx;
all laryngectomees (excluding the severely demented or mentally
retarded) are candidates for an artificial larynx. The question is why
some professionals still do not accept the artificial larynx as a valid communication tool.

When I first started in the area of laryngectomee rehabilitation, two
ideas were stressed: (a) Never refer to esophageal speech as a burp or
belch, and (b) use the artificial larynx only as a last resort. In my opinion,
the application of these concepts was detrimental to laryngectomized
patients.

Paul Scriffignano, executive director of the International Association
of Laryngectomees (IAL) in 1984, wrote "At this year's IAL annual meeting . . . where the theme 'Return to Independence' was brought home
again and again, the message was clear: independence through effective
communication stands as the key to productive, fulfilled lives" (p. 1).

The importance of being able to speak should not have to be
explained or defended. Effective communication is one of the most basic
human needs. We want to speak because of social needs, physical needs,
identity needs, and practical needs. When we are unable to relate to
our environment, we feel a lack of belonging. An inability to communicate means an inability to control, influence, express feelings and desires,
or protect oneself. Denying this ability can affect a person's physical
or mental health and even life itself. This inability reduces what Maslow
(1968) referred to as "self-esteem needs" (the belief that we are worthwhile, deserving people) and "self-actualization" (the belief that we have
potential for improving ourselves).

Yet even today, physicians, social workers, nurses, speech–language pathologists, other laryngectomees, and others deny the laryngectomized patient use of the artificial larynx until other avenues (e.g., esophageal speech) have failed. Then the instrument is offered as a concession of failure. How cruel we sometimes are in our attempts to assist. Marshall Duguay (1978) said,

> Why instead of either esophageal speech or an artificial larynx, can it not be both? Why can't a laryngectomee work on both esophageal speech and artificial larynx speech? Why can't he develop both methods of alaryngeal speech—each to their [sic] fullest extent. (p. 6)

Indeed, why do we hold ourselves responsible for making an either/or choice? As Duguay asked, why not both?

The first time I recall hearing about why the artificial larynx should be used as a primary method of communication was in 1964 at the IAL Voice Institute, Columbia University. This philosophy was expressed by both William Diedrich and Charles Berlin. My own educational and clinical biases caused me to reject this concept for 2 years. Unfortunately, many professionals have retained their biases against devices despite objective data that supports the need for use of speech aids. The literature indicates that 35–60% of laryngectomees will not learn to use esophageal speech, and of those who do, only a small percentage will be rated as good to excellent speakers. If human communication is so important, and I am sure this is doubly so following a laryngectomy, do we have the right to impose biased, sometimes uninformed and misinformed standards for verbal communication on somebody else, particularly a newly laryngectomized patient? Furthermore, no empirical data indicates that learning to use an artificial larynx will interfere with learning to acquire esophageal speech.

In addition to providing a means for immediate oral communication, the following reasons support initial use of an artificial larynx:

1. It may reduce anxiety and tension in the patient and the family, thereby creating a less stressful environment in which to learn esophageal speech.
2. It provides opportunity to practice skills such as compensatory movements for articulation and reduction of stoma noise that must be acquired for production of acceptable esophageal speech.
3. It gives laryngectomees (after some training) viable, understandable speech early in the management process so that effective communication can be used while they are attempting to learn esophageal speech.
4. It is economically beneficial for some patients who must return to work immediately.

5. It reduces both the possibility of acquiring whispered or buccal speech and the need to communicate by writing.
6. It allows individuals who may never be able to use esophageal speech an acceptable method of verbal communication.

Over 100 years ago, Dr. Theodore Christian Billroth performed the first successful laryngectomy for cancer of the larynx. Approximately 21 days later his assistant, Dr. Gussenbauer, designed an artificial larynx for the patient. Since then, many types of artificial larynges have been developed. Why we ever conceived the idea that a person should use an artificial larynx only as a last resort is puzzling. Hopefully, all readers will reject such a negative concept.

INTRODUCING THE ARTIFICIAL LARYNX

It is important that the use of an artificial larynx be introduced early in the postsurgical speech rehabilitation program, ideally while the patient is still in the hospital. The objective is for the individual to begin speaking as soon as possible. The sooner the laryngectomee begins to use oral communication, the more successful will be the total rehabilitation process.

Under most circumstances I do not introduce artificial larynges preoperatively. However, if the family or the patient raises questions regarding such devices, I answer their questions. Generally, preoperative counseling should include information about the services provided by speech pathology and a determination of what the patient and family understand about the impending procedures. Also, the counselor has a chance to learn about the patient and family.

Typically, soon after surgery the clinician introduces the artificial larynx, usually a pneumatic device, an oral adapter on a neck-type device, or an electronic intraoral device. These adapters or devices generally do not interfere with surgical healing unless there has been a complete or partial glossectomy. In addition, they overcome the impedance of surgical dressing, edema, and the presence of a fistula. Patients should be oriented to the device(s) and the clinician should demonstrate use. It behooves clinicians to familiarize themselves with all the instruments and to practice using each for better representation.

Laryngectomees always are informed that each speech aid demonstrated represents a variety of artificial larynx devices. Also, the patients are provided rationale for use of the speech aid at this time—that is, immediate communication until other devices and/or alaryngeal speech methods are considered. Laryngectomees are reminded frequently that learning proper use of the speech aid will prepare them to use other devices and esophageal speech. Patients and family members are instructed how to operate the device, how to change and clean the intra-oral mouth tubes, how and when to change batteries, and how to maintain the instrument. When they are familiar with the speech aid of choice, the clinician provides simple instructions for use.

Prior to being taught specific use of the instrument, the patient is given a routine peripheral speech mechanism examination. One objective is to determine whether the patient wears dentures and, if so, whether they fit properly. Poor-fitting dentures or absence of them can seriously interfere with articulation. Another objective is to determine whether the patient has adequate tongue movement. Reduced tongue movement can interfere with the proper use of the artificial larynx, causing a reduction in intelligibility. Perhaps compensatory movements must be taught. Also, lip mobility is examined. If the patient has any significantly interfering dental, lingual, or lip deviations, it may be wise for the clinician to lower expectations and prepare the patient accordingly.

In addition, an audiological evaluation is conducted. Since most laryngectomees are 50 years of age and older, hearing impairment may be an important variable in (a) deciding which electronic device eventually should be used, and (b) assuring that the patients hear themselves and understand instructions from the clinician.

To this point, procedures for introducing the artificial larynx in a hospital setting have been discussed. Clinicians who do not work in a hospital and see patients only after discharge can follow essentially the same procedures. Indeed, discharged patients will exhibit fewer physical limitations so that the clinician will be able to present and demonstrate a wider variety of devices for selection. If neck-type instruments are demonstrated, the clinician will have to examine carefully the patient's neck for hardness, scar tissue, fistulas, or any other abnormality that would interfere with a proper seal, placement, and vibration of the trans-cervical device.

Immediately after surgery, the patient's selection is limited essentially to a mouth-type device. However, when capable of using a neck-type instrument, the patient should be oriented to all available devices and be encouraged to experiment with them to determine whether to change. The laryngectomee always should make the final choice, with the speech clinician acting as adviser.

The clinician should decide on an individual basis whether to have another laryngectomee present during a patient's orientation and selection process. I decide based on previous experiences and on impressions during the preoperative visit. After deciding that a visiting laryngectomee would be beneficial, the clinician should do the following:

- Discuss the possibility of such a visit with the patient and the family
- Invite a well-rehabilitated laryngectomee who can communicate effectively and use a variety of artificial devices
- Discuss the purpose of the visit with the experienced laryngectomee in advance and clarify the expected role each person will assume in the situation

The importance of introducing the artificial larynx for oral communication as early as possible cannot be overstressed. The clinician and patient thus can begin the rehabilitation process in a very positive way.

INITIAL THERAPY AND THE ARTIFICIAL LARYNX

Intraoral Devices

Essentially the instructions for using an intraoral device are the same regardless of the brand selected. Whether the patient is first introduced to the artificial larynx in the hospital or after discharge, the clinician should follow the same therapy process.

1. Begin by showing, demonstrating, and discussing the various types of intraoral devices. If a pneumatic artificial larynx is going to be used, demonstration by the clinician is impossible. Have a speaker present who uses the pneumatic device or show a videotape. State, or restate, the value of the artificial larynx—that is, that it allows the individual to communicate almost immediately with the clinician, family, employer, friends, and so forth, and that it is complementary to the learning of esophageal speech.

   Demonstrate how the device provides the sound source, and explain that all the laryngectomee must do is articulate. Show how the mouthing of the sounds must be synchronized with activation of the sound source in order to produce the desired speech. Many clinicians speak of a "whispered" sound; however, use of this term sometimes causes patients to exhale air forcefully through the stoma. This stoma noise can mask the artificial larynx speech, thus interfering with the intelligibility of speech.
2. Encourage patients first to operate the various devices without placing the intraoral tube in their mouths.
3. Discuss the following before patients insert the intraoral tube and commence to speak:
   - Handedness—Initially patients will be inclined to operate the artificial larynx with the dominant hand. For years, this was accepted as the most efficient method of operation. Patients have learned,

however, that using the device with the nondominant hand affords them greater use of the dominant hand, for steering a car, shaking hands, or holding a telephone receiver. Therefore, during the initial stages of therapy, the clinician should encourage use of the nondominant hand for operation of the device. However, if this positioning is uncomfortable or if it consistently interferes with the on–off timing, use of the dominant hand is acceptable.

- Placement—Positioning of the intraoral tube can be essential to intelligibility of speech. Users must learn the most comfortable yet most effective placement. In addition, they must be able to achieve accurate placement no less than 90% of the time. Drills for placement can be conducted in conjunction with production of vowel sounds.

When patients first use the mouth-type device, they tend to place the tube directly in the middle of the tongue to produce vowel sounds. To discourage this midline position, the clinician may ask patients to produce a sentence that contains many tongue-tip sounds (e.g., "Tiny Tim tripped 10 times on his teeter–totter"). After attempting to say such a sentence, laryngectomees very quickly become aware that such midline tube placement will interfere greatly with intelligibility.

Blom (1978), Duguay (1983), and Salmon (1978) differ as to how far (¾ in. to 2 in.) the tip of the intraoral tube should be inserted back into a corner of the mouth. Blom suggested, "The mouth tube ... should be placed along the inner lateral surface of the upper first and second molar" (p. 120). This is similar to Duguay's instruction (p. 128). Salmon, on the other hand, instructs the patient to place the tube "into the side of his mouth and to rest it on the upper lateral surface of his tongue" (p. 139). This latter instruction seems much easier for the patient to understand. How far back the tube should be inserted must be determined by each patient's experimentation.

When the patient and clinician have determined the ideal length of tube that should be inserted into the mouth, the distance from the tube tip can be marked with a piece of adhesive tape for the patient to use as a guide to achieve consistent placement. Later, the tape can be removed.

Another idea about placement pertains solely to the pneumatic artificial larynges. The positioning of the mouth tube is the same as previously described; however, the patient also must be concerned with proper coupling of the stoma cup to the tracheostoma. In addition, the clinician should instruct the patient about the need for synchronizing exhalation with phonation and articulation.

Although moderate improvements have been made in the pneumatic-type speech aids, only a small percentage of the laryngectomees in the United States use these devices.

- Blockage—The anterior orifice of the mouth tube can be clogged by saliva or oral and lingual tissue. Patients should be encouraged to experiment with and without the saliva guard on the Cooper-Rand. Some complain that the guard is uncomfortable to hold and that it interferes with flexibility of the mouth tube. To reduce the likelihood of oral or lingual tissue being drawn into the tube opening, the tip of the mouth tube should be cut on a ¼-in. diagonal at a 45° angle. Then the tube should be placed in the mouth with the open side angled upward toward the hard palate. This will reduce clogging of the tube and direct the sound toward the roof of the mouth for better resonance (Salmon, 1983).

- Activation/Deactivation—Generally patients learning to use artificial larynges do one or more of the following: (a) turn the instrument on before placing it in the mouth, (b) start talking with the tube in the mouth before they activate the sound source, or (c) turn the device off before they finish talking.

  The correct timing should be discussed and demonstrated. The best way to practice appropriate timing initially is with vowel production. It is relatively easy to set up a behavioral program. The criterion level the patient must reach should vary between 90% and 100% correct. With almost all patients, this percentage can be achieved during the first therapy session. If the patient is having difficulty with timing, the clinician should audio-record the attempts and elicit patient judgments.

  During the entire process, invite the spouse or any significant other to be present. It is important that they
  —Are aware of the learning process and what is to be expected of the patient.
  —Be trained very early in the therapy program as critical listeners.
  —Be involved in practice at home.
  —Serve as immediate positive reinforcers, under the direction of the clinician.

- Familiarization—The clinician should help the patient and family familiarize themselves with the device. If it is battery operated, they should know where the batteries are located, what kind they are, how they are changed, and so forth. Also, they should know how the tubes are removed, reinserted, and cleaned. All aspects of the care and functioning of the device should be demonstrated. In addition, the patient and family should be "tested" to be sure they understand and are conversant about correct use of the device.

Transcervical Devices

Except for placement, the previously discussed considerations for the mouth-type devices also apply to the neck-type devices.

In placing a transcervical device, the object is to locate the area around the neck that allows for the most efficient coupling of the device to the vocal tract. Since the location varies from patient to patient, placement is usually accomplished by trial and error.

Demonstrate various placements of the device on the neck to illustrate the differences between adequate and inadequate coupling. Encourage the patient to listen to the sounds produced and explain the reasons for the differences perceived. Meanwhile, demonstrate the on–off timing.

The patient must understand that adequate placement is vital to the production of acceptable voice and intelligible speech. An analogy of building a home might be used; without a solid foundation (good placement and timing), the house will surely crumble.

Initially, help the patient achieve the most efficient placement by actually placing the head of the speech aid on various sites of the patient's neck, activating the device, and asking the patient to produce an /a/ sound. Each production should be assessed and discussed until the best location is achieved. Various instruments can be tried in the same manner until the device of choice is determined.

Exact placement of the device is not the only important consideration. Another is the firmness of the vibrating head against the neck site. When proper placement is attained, the appropriate firmness of the seal must be tested through trial and error. If excessive pressure is applied to the site, the vibrations will be dampened, causing poor resonance. Conversely, if too little pressure is applied, sound will escape in the form of extraneous noise and sufficient sound will not be transmitted through the neck and into the oral cavity.

When the correct site and pressure have been established, the site can be marked with a small piece of adhesive tape. The device is then given to the patient, who is instructed to place the instrument on the designated spot. The patient should repeatedly feel for the spot with the empty hand and then place the instrument correctly. Tape is acceptable in the early stages, but must be removed when the patient has a better sense of placement. First the patient is drilled on placement of the device, without sound. When the patient becomes comfortable and feels ready, practice on placement and production of the /a/ begins.

The patient, clinician, and any other listener together should evaluate the production of each sound and determine whether it was good or poor. Such drills will continue until the patient achieves consistent placement and good production of /a/ between 90% and 100% of the time.

The time spent on these drills will vary. Some patients master this skill quickly, whereas others take as long as three ½-hr sessions. When consistent placement and on–off timing of the /a/ sound are excellent, drills on other vowel sounds are conducted.

The significant other is trained to assist the patient with practice at home. The laryngectomee is encouraged to use the artificial larynx at home for answering questions, for making requests, and for general conversation.

When considering electronic devices, the clinician must be concerned with the patient's and listener's hearing abilities. Since most of these people are 50 years of age or older, presbycusis (a bilateral hearing loss with the high frequencies affected first) should be suspected.

Certainly a significant hearing loss will affect the person's ability to successfully learn to use an electronic device. Because of the noise factors inherent in the electronic devices, the signal-to-noise ratio may mask the hearing that does exist. Patients' inability to monitor their own speech will interfere with learning. Listeners' inability to hear the speech will interfere with understanding.

Assume that the patient has a bilateral hearing loss and is wearing two hearing aids. If a neck-type artificial larynx is being used, the noise produced by the device can drive the hearing aids to their maximum level and severely distort the output. If the patient has only one hearing aid, it is suggested that the artificial larynx be used on the opposite side. Although some distortion will continue, it may not be as severe as it would be if the device were placed on the side where the hearing aid is located. In either case, it might be advisable to adjust the device to as low a pitch as possible. This adjustment should improve self-monitoring skills. Another possibility, especially with patients wearing bilateral aids, is to explore the use of current hearing aid technology to reduce the level of background noise, particularly in the low frequencies. The point is that clinicians should be aware of the patient's and listener's hearing abilities and, if a hearing loss exists, should seek a speech aid compatible with a hearing aid that will offer the best opportunity for self-monitoring and understanding.

Continued Therapy

We clinicians receive a great feeling of satisfaction when patients master placement and timing and begin to produce longer speech units. Thus we sometimes reduce the effort that might be directed toward further therapy. We fool ourselves by thinking that, following limited instruction, the patients will be capable of learning on their own. This is certainly not the case. If ratings of intelligibility are dependent on articulation, then continued articulation drill is necessary. Practice on consonants is more important than on vowels. Consonant drill should start with consonant–vowel (CV) production and proceed through VCV, words, short phrases, and so on. Goldstein (1978) stated, "Unfortunately there is a tendency among clinicians and laryngectomees to slow down the rate of speech and to over-articulate when using a device. This tendency decreases intelligibility by distorting the inherent rhythm of language" (p. 129).

I both disagree and agree with this statement. Some stuttering programs recommend reducing the rate of speech while drilling on consonant production to improve self-monitoring. This technique may be equally useful to laryngectomees. Conversely, Goldstein's statement in regard to overarticulation seems reasonable. When the concept of correct articulation, particularly that of final consonants, is achieved, the clinician should encourage patients to use their normal rate. With individuals who exhibited no speech problems prior to surgery and who presently have adequate functioning of the articulators, such work usually does not exceed two sessions.

In addition to articulation and rate, the concept of phrasing also should be stressed. Some clinicians (Blom, 1978; Duguay, 1983) recommend the phrasing exercises used in the drillbook by Fairbanks (1959). These exercises should be tape-recorded to allow patients to monitor themselves. Drills of this type usually do not exceed more than one or two sessions.

Many clinicians (Blom 1978; Duguay, 1983; Goldstein, 1978; Salmon, 1983) have stressed the need for patients to produce distinctions between voiced and voiceless consonants. I tend to be more concerned with what I shall refer to as "context intelligibility." It seems logical that during everyday speech, the redundancy of the language and the contextual cues will, for the most part, overcome the voiced/voiceless confusions. However, when drill on this aspect is necessary, the focus should be primarily on initial and final sounds in a phrase. These drills also require proper on–off timing, which was taught to the patient in the initial speech sessions.

Awareness of context intelligibility is best gained through a group therapy situation. The patient can either read something or relate an incident. Then the group members are asked whether they understood what was said and are asked to repeat it.

ADVANCED THERAPY

Far too often clinicians tend to discontinue artificial larynx speech therapy as they attempt to help patients develop esophageal sound. If the patients are unable to achieve esophageal speech, clinicians often do not return to therapy with the artificial larynx. Unless patients insist, therapy with the artificial larynx should not be discontinued until they acquire speech that is relatively normal sounding. This means there is a need to work on such aspects as pitch, inflection, and consistent use of the device outside the clinic and within the home environment.

Because of their electromechanical features, most artificial larynges produce a single pitch, monotonous tone, and specified loudness. In other words, once the pitch and loudness controls are set, they cannot be changed during running speech. The exceptions are the pneumatic devices and the new Servox Inton.

Patients using the pneumatic device can learn to actively change some aspects of loudness and pitch through control of their own pulmonary functioning. This control can be taught through experimentation during the therapy process.

The frequency control button on the Western Electric #5A or #5B could be manipulated to achieve pitch variability. This feature no longer exists, however, in the newer #5C model. The Servox Inton is designed for adjustment of the fundamental frequency and for adjustment of pitch during speech production by using the two control buttons. The upper button can be used to produce the basic pitch, whereas activation of the lower button produces a sound one-half tone higher in pitch than that of the top button. The manufacturer states that patients can learn to use these buttons appropriately to add inflection and intonation to their speech.

I have instructed a few patients in the use of the Servox Inton. It takes time and training to learn proper manipulation of the two control buttons. For their patients' sake, all clinicians should learn to use the control buttons by practicing the drills suggested in the instruction manual. In addition, they should use the device with fellow colleagues to determine whether they are using the buttons to achieve correct intonation patterns. Older patients have exhibited difficulty with these button manipulations. Also, the majority of patients resort to the use of their dominant hand to better control the two maneuvers. Despite these drawbacks, this mechanical innovation by DR. Kuhn & Co. is encouraging.

The other neck-type devices are not designed for any mechanical control or change of pitch during conversation. Minor pitch changes can be obtained, however, by altering the coupling pressure of the instrument on the neck. Changes in the coupling can be carried out by starting with production of vowels, then single words, and finally short phrases. In addition, stress can be achieved by instructing patients to use longer duration and slightly higher pitch. Utilizing such drills for intonation and stress will help develop the prosodic features of speech. Although some patients achieve these skills without training, most must be taught.

Few authors discuss the need for "situational therapy" (see Duguay, 1983). Many laryngectomees use their devices only in limited environments such as home and the speech clinic. Therefore, it is important that clinicians encourage use of the artificial larynx in a wide variety of settings. Patients should be encouraged to establish a hierarchy of situations they consider the easiest or least threatening to the most difficult. Duguay (1983) offered some excellent suggestions for activities that might be introduced during this phase of treatment. Clinicians should be present during the initial activities, but as the patients gain confidence, clinicians can encourage more independent practice.

TROUBLE-SHOOTING THE ARTIFICIAL LARYNX

The purchase of an artificial larynx represents a substantial financial investment. To protect this investment and to obtain the most beneficial and efficient use, care and maintenance of the device is required. Some practicable suggestions for the patient are listed below.

- Do not abuse the device by banging or dropping it. When not in use, make sure the device is kept in a pocket or other receptacle where it will not be damaged.
- Do not leave an electronic device exposed to excessive moisture. None of these devices is guaranteed for moisture damage.
- Make sure the instrument is turned off when not in use.
- Check the device each morning before using it to note any changes in its functioning.

Like all mechanical devices, the artificial larynx is subject to malfunction and breakdown. This will cause concern on the part of the laryngectomee and family; however, a great deal of this concern can be avoided when both the patient and the family are well acquainted with the device and how it functions.

A variety of mechanical difficulties may occur. The suggestions listed below may prove helpful to both clinicians and patients.

If the cause of the difficulty cannot be determined, the device should be returned to the manufacturer. Under no circumstances should the device be taken apart in an attempt to manipulate the internal mechanism.

Problem	Possible cause
	Pneumatic Larynx
Not producing sound	• Plugged tubing (Tube should be cleaned daily) • Leak in system • Vibrating reed may be malfunctioning • Poor stoma seal
	Electronic Larynx
Not producing sound	• Dead or discharged battery (An inexpensive battery tester can be purchased at most electronic stores. Patients should always keep a spare battery with them. Remove battery each night.) • Battery placed in the reverse position (Plus and minus signs should be lined up on both battery and battery compartment) • Wrong type of battery (Check instruction manual) • Loose-fitting battery (On certain models the battery must be placed in tightly, as in a flashlight) • Battery contacts corroded (These should be cleaned periodically with fine sandpaper) • Broken cord (If device has a cord, examine for breaks or inadequate contact) • Off–on switch may be defective (This will require factory service) • Intraoral transducer is damaged from excessive moisture
Sound is weak	• Weak battery • Poor battery contacts • Malfunction of the volume control button • Poor internal control of the vibrator in the neck-type devices • Cord is plugged in backward so that impedance is mismatched
Intermittent sound	• Weak battery • Corroded battery contacts • Broken cord or poor contact • Malfunctioning volume or pitch control

REFERENCES

Barney, H. L. (1958). A discussion of some technical aspects of speech aids for postlaryngectomized patients. *Annals of Otology, Rhinology and Laryngology, 67,* 558–570.

Barney, H. L., Haworth, F. E., & Dunn, H. K. (1959). An experimental transistorized artificial larynx. *Bell System Technical Journal, 38,* 1337–1356.

Blom, E. D. (1978). The artificial larynx: Past and present. In S. J. Salmon & L. P. Goldstein (Eds.), *The artificial larynx handbook* (pp. 57–86). New York: Grune and Stratton.

Blom, E. D. (1979). The artificial larynx: Types and modifications. In R. L. Keith & F. L. Darley (Eds.), *Laryngectomee rehabilitation* (pp. 63–86). Austin, TX: PRO-ED.

Czermak, J. (1859). Über die Sprache bei luftdichter Verschliessung des Kehlkopfes. Sitzungesberichte der Akademie der Wessenschaften in Wien. *Mathematisch-naturiuessenschaftliche Klasse, 35,* 65–72.

Duguay, M. (1978). Why not both? In S. J. Salmon & L. P. Goldstein (Eds.), *The artificial larynx handbook* (pp. 3–10). New York: Grune & Stratton.

Duguay, M. (1983). Teaching use of an artificial larynx. In W. H. Perkins (Ed.), *Voice disorders* (pp. 127–130). New York: Thieme-Stratton.

Fairbanks, G. (1959). *Voice and articulation drillbook.* New York: Harper.

Goldstein, L. P. (1978). Approaches to treatment: Part D. In S. J. Salmon & L. P. Goldstein (Eds.), *The artificial larynx handbook* (pp. 127–129). New York: Grune and Stratton.

Greene, J. S. (1942a). Composite postoperative therapy for the laryngectomized. *Medical World, 60,* 115.

Greene, J. S. (1942b). Rehabilitating the laryngectomized patient. *Bulletin of the American Society of Cancer, 24,* 5.

Gussenbauer, C. (1874). Über die erste durch Billroth am Menschen ausgeführte Kehlkopf—Extirpation und die Anwendung eines kunstlichen Kehlkopfes. *Archiv für die klinische chirurgie, 17,* 343–356.

Lebrun, Y. (1973). The artificial larynx. *Neurolinguistics.* Amsterdam: Swet and Zeitlinger.

Lowry, L. D. (1981). Artificial larynges: A review and development of a prototype self-contained intra-oral artificial larynx. *Laryngoscope, 91,* 1332–1355.

Maslow, A. H. (1968). *Toward a psychology of being.* New York: Van Nostrand, Reinhold.

Salmon, S. J. (1978). Approaches to treatment: Part F. In S. J. Salmon & L. P. Goldstein (Eds.), *The artificial larynx handbook* (pp. 137–144). New York: Grune and Stratton.

Salmon, S J. (1983). Artificial larynx speech: A viable means of alaryngeal communication. In Y. Edels (Ed.), *Laryngectomy: Diagnosis to rehabilitation* (pp. 142–162). London: Croom Helm.

Salmon, S. J., & Goldstein, L. P. (Eds.). (1978). *The artificial larynx handbook.* New York: Grune and Stratton.

Scriffignano, P. (1984, Summer/Fall). Speaking out. *IAL News,* p. 1.

Weinberg, B. (1981). Speech alteration following total laryngectomy. In J. R. Darby (Ed.), *Speech evaluation in medicine* (pp. 128–158). New York: Grune and Stratton.

CHAPTER 3

Esophageal Speech Training: The Initial Phase

Marshall J. Duguay

> *Duguay's tutorial provides a step-by-step approach to initial esophageal voice training. He anticipates patients' behaviors that may occur during the treatment process and suggests various approaches that can be used to reinforce or diminish them, setting as his goal the documentation of procedures for teaching patients to acquire excellent esophageal speech.*

Study Questions

1. Why do the consonants /p/, /t/, and /k/ facilitate esophageal air intake for alaryngeal speech?
2. Which method of air intake is preferred for esophageal phonation?
3. When esophageal phonation is established and consistent, what is the next goal in therapy?

The purpose of this chapter is to enable the reader who has only limited familiarity with esophageal speech to attend his or her first postlaryngectomy speech session possessing a clear understanding of the mechanics of esophageal phonation, the goals, and the way to proceed.

The profession of speech–language pathology offers innumerable challenges and rewards. I am especially enamored with the area of patient contact. Observing the patient's first production of esophageal voice is truly an extraordinary experience.

When one watches a great surgeon, athlete, artist, or, for that matter, a great anything, one is always impressed with how easy the task looks. The apparent ease may be misleading because much preparation, thought, and training had to precede the witnessed event. The clinician needs to undergo this same preparation prior to the therapy session designed to initiate esophageal phonation. This preparation, very much like our profession, is part art and part science.

PHONATORY SITE

Diedrich and Youngstrom (1966) wrote,

> Esophageal speech is that in which the vicarious air chamber is located within the lumen of the esophagus and the neoglottis is located above (cephalad) the air chamber. The site of the neoglottis is the pharyngoesophageal (PE) segment or junction, and may contain fibers of the inferior constrictor, cricopharyngeus, and/or the superior esophageal sphincter which are predominantly located at [cervical vertebra 5 (C5)] and C6. (p. 108)

The term *neoglottis* is used by Decroix, Libersa, and Lattard (1958) and by Diedrich and Youngstrom (1966) to signify a new glottis. As one reviews the radiographic studies of Damsté (1958), Hodson and Oswald (1958), and Vrticka and Svoboda (1961), one cannot help but be impressed by the striking variability of neoglottic sites (see Figure 3.1). Since the sites are variable, Diedrich and Youngstrom (1966) referred to the vibratory site as the *pharyngoesophageal (PE) segment,* a term that will be used throughout this chapter.

AIR CHARGING

To power the PE segment for esophageal phonation, the air present in the oropharyngeal cavity must twice transgress (air in–sound out) this normally closed barrier rapidly and with ease. Laryngectomized individuals must learn something motorically different from swallowing if they hope to achieve rapid, fluent, and completely normal-appearing esophageal speech. The complex and cumbersome patterns associated

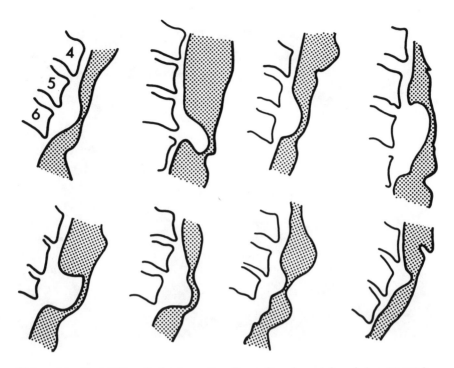

Figure 3.1. Variability of vibratory sites. From *Oesophageal Speech* (pp. 38–39) by P. H. Damsté, 1958, Groningen, The Netherlands: Boekdrukkerij Voorheen Gerroeders Hoitsema. Reprinted by permission of P. H. Damsté.

with swallowing are completely different from those associated with fluent esophageal speech. The muscles used in swallowing cannot be fired and then recover quickly for most speakers to achieve effortless esophageal speech. Consequently, instructing a patient to swallow or to drink carbonated beverages should be used only as a last resort, a desperation technique in therapy. If readers doubt the severe limitation of swallowing, then they are invited to swallow four or five times in rapid succession. It cannot be done.

The upper third of the esophagus can be charged with air using one or both methods of air intake commonly referred to as *air injection* or *air inhalation*. A detailed explanation of these methods appears later in this chapter. For now, consider a simplified analogy of making sound with a toy balloon to understand the extremely complex process of esophageal phonation. First, picture a balloon in a collapsed state (Figure 3.2). To inflate the balloon, one must force air through a narrow opening. To make sound, one also needs to apply the "correct" amount of

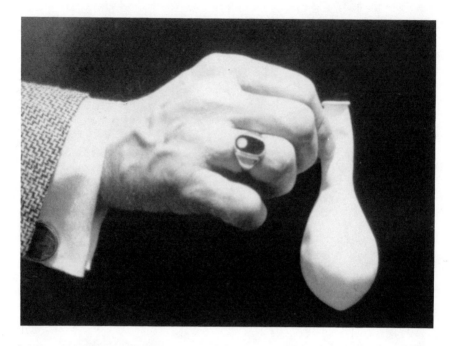

Figure 3.2. Collapsed balloon.

pressure at the neck of the balloon and slowly release some of the air. The voluntary release of air, combined with the inherent elasticity of the balloon, will move air through the narrowed region and cause this portion of the balloon to vibrate and produce sound (Figure 3.3).

Creating sound with a balloon requires the precise interaction of three pressure systems. We need to blow air into the balloon (Pressure System 1) from a source superior to the region where the fingers grasp it. If we grasp the balloon too tightly with our fingers (Pressure System 2), air cannot enter it. Once air is in the balloon, too tight a grip will prevent air from exiting; too loose a grip will cause the air to escape without the production of noticeable sound. Finally, air is forced back out of the balloon (Pressure System 3) by the collapse of the elastic-like walls of the balloon.

One can use the balloon analogy to understand the balanced and dynamic relationship that must occur among three pressure systems to produce esophageal phonation. The pressure systems involved in esophageal sound production are represented in Figure 3.4. Pressure System 1 is the normal atmospheric pressure that is present in the

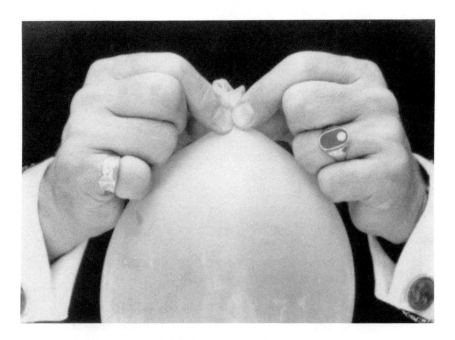

Figure 3.3. Sound production with a balloon.

oropharyngeal cavity, superior to the PE segment. Pressure System 2 is the muscular, tonic resistance of the normally closed PE segment, the vibratory site. Pressure System 3 is the air pressure in the normally semicollapsed esophagus itself, inferior to the PE segment. Remember that esophageal pressure is less than atmospheric pressure in the oropharyngeal cavity. Intraesophageal pressure has been measured at readings from −4 to −7 mm Hg (Atkinson, Kramer, Wyman, & Inglefinger, 1957; Dey & Kirchner, 1961).

Figure 3.5 juxtaposes the balloon and esophageal sound production systems. To create sound, the esophagus must be charged with the oropharyngeal air supply, and then the air must be quickly expelled to set the PE segment into vibration. Also, it is important to recognize that although the esophagus is continuous with the stomach, the oropharyngeal air introduced into the esophagus should never enter the stomach. Superior esophageal phonation, as stated earlier, is accomplished in a manner other than swallowing air into the stomach and then belching it back out. Thus, it is advisable to avoid using the terms *swallow* and *belch* when working with a laryngectomized patient, since

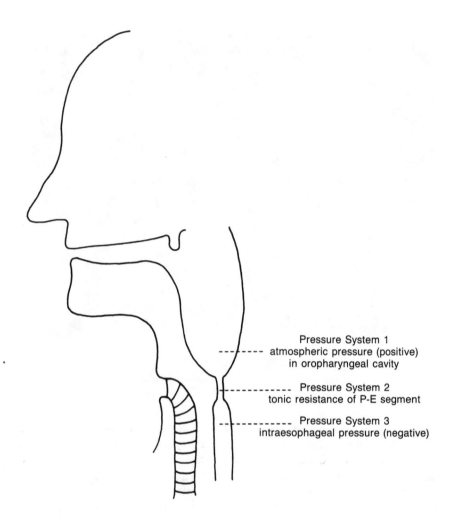

Figure 3.4. The three pressure systems used in esophageal phonation.

he or she may conjure behaviors that are in opposition to the appropriate methods of air intake and expulsion required for esophageal phonation. The obvious question, then, is if one does not swallow air into the esophagus, how does one load or charge it with the available oropharyngeal air supply? The answer is by air injection and/or air inhalation. Although these two methods can coexist, they are discussed separately to facilitate understanding.

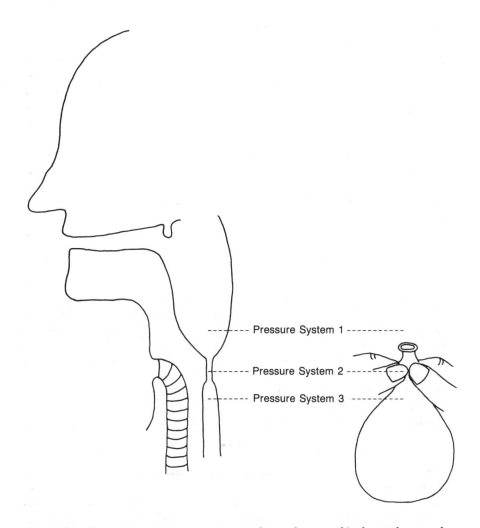

Figure 3.5. Comparison of pressure systems used to produce sound in the esophagus and with a balloon.

Air Charging Via Injection Methods

The ability to achieve air intake via the injection method requires adaptations to Pressure System 1, the oropharyngeal air pressure. Injection demands that oropharyngeal pressure be sufficiently increased to override the muscular, tonic pressure keeping the PE segment closed. The oropharyngeal air can then enter and inflate the semicollapsed esophagus (filling the balloon). How can oropharyngeal air pressure be increased? By decreasing the size of the oropharyngeal cavity, the air molecules are forced into a smaller space, thus increasing pressure. With the injection technique, the size of the space in the oropharyngeal cavity is reduced by movements of the tongue, lips, cheeks, and pharynx. These movements serve to compress the air that is present in the oropharyngeal cavity into a smaller space, providing a pressure buildup sufficient to override and force open the PE segment, thus "injecting" air into the esophagus. To develop a successful pressure buildup, two of the three exits for air to escape from the oropharyngeal cavity must be closed. The air present in the mouth and throat can escape through the lips, through the nose, or down into the esophagus. Since the goal is to move air into the esophagus from the mouth and throat, the patient must (a) close off the nasal port via velopharyngeal closure and (b) close off the oral port via a lip and/or tongue seal.

Tongue Injection. Movements of the tongue utilized to decrease cavity size and hence increase oropharyngeal pressure, fall into two distinct but related patterns. These movement patterns are described by Diedrich and Youngstrom (1966) as either a glossal press or a glossopharyngeal press. According to Diedrich and Youngstrom, during a glossal press the tongue tip contacts the alveolar ridge, and frequently the middle of the tongue contacts the hard and soft palates. The posterior portion of the tongue makes a backward movement, but does not actually touch the posterior wall. Velopharyngeal closure must occur to prevent nasal air escape. Oral air escape can be prevented by lip closure, although this is not necessary since the tongue provides the primary seal for the oral port (see Figure 3.6).

During a glossopharyngeal press the tip and middle portion of the tongue are in contact with the alveolus, hard palate, and soft palate. The posterior portion of the tongue moves backward and actually contacts the posterior pharyngeal wall. Sometimes, contact is enhanced by pharyngeal wall movement. Similar to the glossal press, velopharyngeal closure occurs and the oral port is sealed with the tongue or lips (see Figure 3.7). It is preferable to accomplish oral port closure by using the tongue rather than the lips during both glossal and glossopharyngeal presses. The reasons for this preference should become apparent in the following discussion about lip injection.

Lip Injection. Instead of using the tongue to compress, squeeze, and hence inject air into the esophagus, it is possible to use buccal and pharyngeal musculature to contract the oropharyngeal cavity. The process is similar to puffing up the cheeks with air and pushing on them with the fingers while keeping the lips tightly sealed. Instead of forcing the air through the lips, the compression "squirts" the air backward

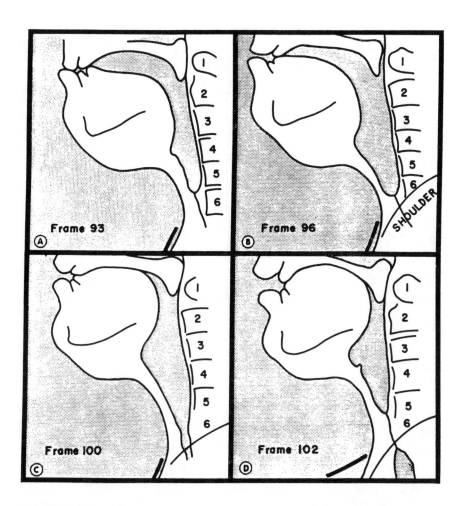

Figure 3.6. The glossal press method of air injection. From *Alaryngeal Speech* (p. 39) by W. M. Diedrich and K. A. Youngstrom, 1966, Springfield, IL: Charles C. Thomas. Reprinted by permission.

and down into the esophagus. With this lip injection technique, the lips, cheeks, and pharynx contract to reduce the cavity size, thereby increasing the pressure and overriding the tonic closure of the PE segment. Another way to conceptualize this technique is to imagine holding your breath while saying the phoneme /p/, but forcing the air backward rather than forward in the usual manner.

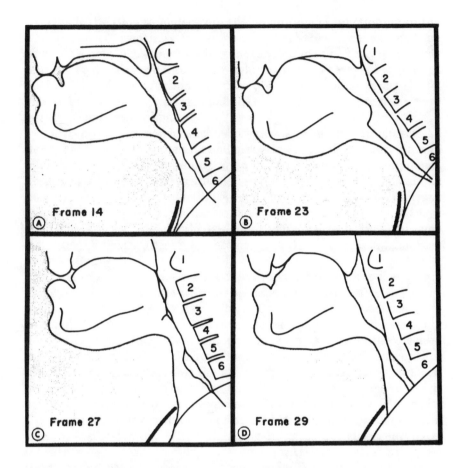

Figure 3.7. The glossopharyngeal press method of air injection. From *Alaryngeal Speech* (p. 40) by W. M. Diedrich and K. A. Youngstrom, 1966, Springfield, IL: Charles C. Thomas. Reprinted by permission.

The lip injection technique has a cosmetic drawback. The pursing and squeezing movements of the lips to inject air are distracting. Speech needs to look good as well as sound good, and lip injection does not enhance visual communication. Parenthetically, one might hypothesize that the erroneous and old-fashioned belief that one swallows air to produce esophageal voice arose because of the similarity between the lip postures seen during swallowing and lip injection.

If patients who use lip injection have distracting lip mannerisms, it is important to convert them to tongue injection. A useful technique to prevent the lips from coming together is to place a pencil or pen sideways in the mouth between the second or third molars. This obstruction forces use of the tongue for the injection maneuver.

The "Dutch Method" of Air Injection (Consonant Injection). A substantial body of literature exists that apparently started with the writings of Moolenaar-Bijl (1953a, 1953b) and Damsté (1958). In these early articles they discussed the use of plosive consonants to facilitate injection of air. Because these writers are from the Netherlands, consonant injection is sometimes referred to as the "Dutch method." The plosive sounds generate an oropharyngeal pressure buildup that can overcome the PE segment barrier to the esophagus. The plosives most frequently used for this facilitating maneuver are /p, t, k/. The associated motor movements of these loading consonants can be used to inject air. The three motor patterns associated with these phonemes are similar to those described for the three methods of air injection. The motor pattern for the phoneme /t/ is the glossal press, for /k/ the glossopharyngeal press (the two types of tongue injection), and for /p/ the oropharyngeal press (lip injection). Other pressure consonants such as /s, ʃ, tʃ, dʒ/ can be used to attain air injection.

Air Charging Via the Inhalation Method

The major differences between air inhalation and air injection are in how the esophagus is inflated and how the PE segment opens. Recall that intraesophageal pressure readings register around −4 to −7 mm Hg relative to atmospheric pressure (Atkinson et al., 1957; Dey & Kirchner, 1961). Inhalation of air from the oropharynx through the PE segment and into the esophagus is accomplished by further decreasing the negative esophageal pressure. The positive air pressure from the mouth and throat will flow to the negative air pressure in the esophagus. To further decrease the negative intraesophageal air pressure, the laryngectomized person needs only to inhale pulmonary air through the tracheostoma. Inhalation will accomplish a pressure drop in the esophagus that can reach levels as low as −10, −15, or −20 mm Hg. As a direct result of the pressure differential between Pressure System 1 and Pressure System 3, air is "sucked" into the esophagus *if* the tonic closure of the PE segment is not too great. A precise balance between the three pressure systems is critical to accomplish successful esophageal insufflation (see Figure 3.8). Failure in any one of the three systems can produce adverse effects on the overall process of esophageal phonation.

Unlike injection, inhalation does not require an increase in air pressure by compression of cavity size, so sealing off the oral and/or velopharyngeal ports is unnecessary. However, many patients actually do close off one or both ports.

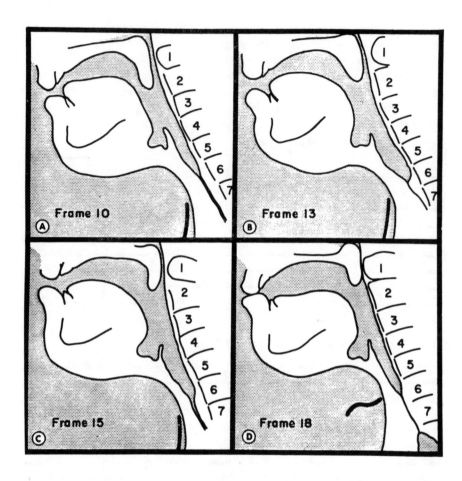

Figure 3.8. The inhalation method of air intake for esophageal phonation. From *Alaryngeal Speech* (p. 38) by W. M. Diedrich and K. A. Youngstrom, 1966, Springfield, IL: Charles C. Thomas. Reprinted by permission.

Although the two methods of air intake are discussed separately, their use is not mutually exclusive and may coexist in the same speaker. In the majority of speakers who employ both methods of air intake, however, one of the methods assumes a primary role. Also, a patient who uses an injection method of air charging can use one, two, or all three methods of air injection, often as a response to the articulatory demands of the utterance. Diedrich and Youngstrom (1966) indicated that esophageal speech skill is not related to the method of air intake utilized by a speaker. Recent personal communications with J. C. Shanks

(November 11, 1988) and N. T. Donnelly (October 5, 1988) reinforce my long-held belief that cultural and linguistic differences may partially account for the type of air intake used. The majority of Japanese and Chinese speakers employ inhalation as their primary method of air intake, whereas the majority of Americans use primarily injection methods.

EXPELLING ESOPHAGEAL AIR FOR PHONATION

The principles by which esophageal speakers expel the injected and/or inhaled air from the esophagus are not as well understood as are the dynamics of air charging. The concept of synchrony between pulmonary air expulsion and esophageal phonation is supported by the work of DiCarlo, Amster, and Herer (1956); Motta, Profazio, and Acciarri (1959); Robe, Moore, Andrews, and Holinger (1956); Schlosshauer and Mockel (1958); Snidecor and Isshiki (1965); and, to some extent, Diedrich and Youngstrom (1966). Although Diedrich and Youngstrom (1966) found evidence to support synchrony, they also reported behaviors that contradict it. Rapid acquisition of esophageal phonation following laryngectomy lends support to synchronization of this lifelong behavior of exhalation–phonation. Also, most esophageal speakers exhibit behaviors consistent with coordination of respiration and phonation.

Factors accounting for esophageal air expulsion include resistance of the PE segment, intraesophageal pressures, tonus and elasticity of the esophageal walls, and extrinsic adjustments of pulmonary esophageal pressure through muscle tension and contraction. As air is expelled, an extremely rapid reduction of total esophageal diameter, almost a collapse, appears to move from the region of the distal or cardiac sphincter upward toward the proximal or PE segment (Damsté, 1958).

INITIATING ESOPHAGEAL SOUND

Whenever possible, the clinician should establish a relationship and rapport with the patient prior to the initial session planned to evoke esophageal sound. The relationship can be developed through pre- and postoperative counseling, hospital visitations, and/or instruction in the use of an artificial larynx. I have long been an avid proponent of a dual approach to postlaryngectomy speech (Duguay, 1968, 1978, 1986).

Esophageal voice therapy can begin as soon as the nasogastric feeding tube has been removed, approximately 7 to 10 days after surgery. If a small fistula is present, the clinician should consult with the physician since voice therapy may need to be delayed until complete healing has been accomplished. When medical clearance has been obtained, esophageal speech training can commence. A delay in starting voice therapy should not be any hardship on the patient because he or she should have been talking with an artificial larynx since surgery.

When the clinician approaches the first session to evoke sound, he or she should have two goals in mind, only one of which is shared with the patient. The clinician's goal is to have the patient leave that session with the ability to say several words using his or her new esophageal voice. However, if the patient knows the goal is to develop sound and speech at the first session, he or she may feel pressure to achieve that goal. That pressure may engender anxiety and tension in the region of the PE segment. Too much tension can cause the PE segment to become so resistant that air charging becomes virtually impossible. The pressure should be felt by the clinician, not by the patient. The patient should believe that the goal is to experiment and to try a few things to make sound.

Clinicians should create an atmosphere that is comfortable, relaxed, and supportive. They need to appear confident and assured. Years of study and training and the very favorable odds of achieving success at this initial phonation session are all positive factors. Also, many patients who arrive for the initial esophageal speech session already are creating sound and using esophageal speech. This ability may exist at a volitional level, or it may be a behavior that is emitted nonvolitionally. The clinician's first order of business is to discover whether esophageal phonation is an ability the patient brings to this initial session. Good teacher–clinicians are more leaders than teachers. Consequently, before clinicians have to teach, they should find out what abilities the patients have and lead them from there.

Indirect Methods

Begin by asking whether the patient can say any words or make any sounds without using the speech aid. Can he or she make that sound or say that word now or remember what the word was that just "popped out"? Clinicians will be amazed at the number of patients who will begin using esophageal speech. When this occurs, carefully observe the precise behaviors employed. What method of air intake is used? Are any consonants facilitating air charging? Is the patient an inhaler, tongue injector, lip injector, or a combination of these? Also, listen for any evidence or sign of air going into the esophagus. Perhaps the patient demonstrates no esophageal phonation, but may be loading air inconsistently. The clinician's ability to critically listen and identify air going in or sound coming out is the major clinical skill required at this point. Clinicians need to know how the patient is insufflating air. For example, the patient who is able to say the word "tie" is probably a tongue injector and is employing glossal press. Ask him or her to say "tie" several times. Then ask the patient to say other words beginning with /t/. To take advantage of the successful CV base, select stimulus words that have the vowel /aɪ/ as in the word "tie," such as, "time," "tight," and "tile." Obviously, the same protocol would be followed for words beginning with /p, k, tʃ, ʃ, dʒ/. If the patient "says" he or she cannot make any sound, add some nonspeech sounds for the patient to imitate. The word "says" is used because it is desirable to have the patient "talk" and reply without the device while the clinician "speech reads" and carefully listens for clues of air in or sound out. Try things like the "tsk, tsk" of scolding, the sound some make to call a cat, the "giddyap" sound to a horse, the raspberry or Bronx cheer used to express dislike, spitting tobacco, and even the oral sound some children employ to mimic the expulsion of flatus. Let your clinical imagination and creativity add to this sound list and employ sounds of your childhood, region, and culture. Listen intently for any "kickback" of air from a loading consonant into the esophagus. Also, be sure to have the patient say the sound as loudly as possible to generate higher intraoral pressures. Accept any excess stoma noise that may occur along with the extra effort expended to "talk louder." The stoma blast obviously will need to be minimized as soon as it is clinically feasible.

If you hear any esophageal phonation or the sound of air entering the esophagus, (a) stop the patient, (b) identify the sound, and (c) have the patient repeat the behavior that caused the sound. Have the patient do this a number of times until the sound becomes consistent. Directions should be simple. If any sound of air entering the esophagus is identified, say something like, "Right there I heard a tiny sound in your throat. Do that again. That's it! Do it again. That's it. Again!" At this point, do not stop to examine the behavior. Drill more and more before trying to figure out exactly what is causing the result. Do not intellectualize the process at this point. There are too many things to analyze, and calling attention to the process now can change order or cause tension and result in failure. The clinician's role at this point is that of a cheerleader: "That's it. Again! Once more. Again! Once more." After the behavior that evokes sound is consistent and established, it often is helpful to have the patient label or describe what he or she is doing to make sound. Even if the response is incorrect in terms of clinical knowledge of esophageal phonation, it becomes an appropriate stimulus label for the behavior and has a semantic value for the patient. For example, if the patient describes the behavior as "half a swallow," use the descriptive label as a stimulus for evoking sound by saying, "Give me half a swallow and produce _____."

If no sound has been produced volitionally, continue talking with the patient by taking a modified case history or inquiring about family, work, hobbies, and so forth. This additional interaction provides more time to listen for any indication of air entering or exiting the esophagus and to identify, reinforce, and develop that available behavior. The sound of air entering the esophagus has been aptly described by Diedrich and Youngstrom (1966) as "klunking." The klunk may be quite loud or barely audible. Acoustically, but not behaviorally, it is similar to the audible gulp one hears when swallowing. The klunk indicates that air has entered the esophagus and is immediately available for rapid return to create esophageal phonation. If the klunk is heard during conversation, it signals the halfway point toward esophageal phonation since the air now available needs only to be returned in order to phonate. When the clinician hears or the patient "feels" this klunk, the patient should immediately try to say a vowel or a simple VC word, such as "up," "at," or "ate," as *quickly* and *loudly* as possible. Quick production prevents the air from moving down into the stomach from which retrieval is difficult, and loud production employs abdominal and extrinsic forces needed to drive air out of the esophagus. Accept any klunking and/or stoma blasts that occur at this time. If necessary, reassure the patient that at some later date these two behaviors will need to be extinguished.

If the sound of air either entering (klunk) or leaving (phonation) has not been heard after a reasonable amount of time has been invested in these activities, try the following suggestion. Ask the patient to repeat as loudly as possible a sound or word that is initiated with a loading consonant: "tuh, tuh, tuh," or "puh, puh, puh," or "kuh, kuh, kuh," or "tie, tie, tie." Other words to repeat include "tip," "taught," "talk," "pop," "pep," "pie," "pip," "cake," "kick," and "kite." If sound (air in or sound out) occurs on a word that has two possible but different loading consonants, such as the word "kite," be sure to identify whether one or both consonants were helpful in loading air. Also, be extremely careful when using /k/ loaded words that what you hear and reinforce in terms of sound production is esophageal speech and not pharyngeal speech as described in chapter 1. Do not reinforce pharyngeal sound, which is created within the pharyngeal area above a PE segment that is tightly closed.

When consistency of phonation has been established, begin to identify the behaviors employed to achieve air in and sound out. The patient needs to understand explicitly what he or she is doing to create sound so that he or she can learn to control the act. The patient should not "just try" and hope that sound is produced, but rather should know that if he or she does a particular "thing," he or she can load air for esophageal speech. It is important that the patient be aware of both the feel and the sound of air entering the esophagus. The patient can place a hand to the throat and actually feel the air entering the esophagus; or the patient can hear the sound when it is amplified via a tape recorder after the microphone has been placed on the throat. Cues such as these help the patient develop volitional control of phonation. Obtaining nonvolitional sound is relatively easy. Acquiring control of that sound is what therapy accomplishes through a systematic progression of exercises and activities.

Semidirect Method

Several behaviors can be employed to inject or to inhale air into the esophagus. A number of these behaviors include postures that are clearly observable. The underlying principle of the semidirect method is to combine all of these behaviors into a visible and acoustic model. The clinician presents the composite model and observes which behavior(s) the patient "selects" for loading air. The model should combine behaviors representative of those observed in inhalation, tongue injection, lip injection, and the Dutch method. The person who uses inhalation frequently employs a sniffing motion, an upward and outward thrust of the mandible, and an open mouth. The injector uses the tongue, closes the mouth, and evidences some lip pursing and pharyngeal contraction. An individual who uses the Dutch method employs the consonant sounds /p/, /t/, and /k/.

To model these behaviors, begin with an open mouth, then sniff, jut the mandible outward and upward, raise the tongue tip to the alveolar ridge, close the mouth, squeeze the lips and throat, and say /tʌ/. Repeat the entire model and say /pʌ/. Then repeat the entire model but end with saying /kʌ/. Ask the patient to watch and then after each presentation copy exactly what he or she saw. Careful monitoring of the patient's attempts is necessary to determine which of the behaviors facilitated loading of air. Did the air enter when the patient sniffed and raised the chin (inhalation), when the tongue went up to the alveolar ridge (tongue injection), when the lips closed (lip injection), or when he or she attempted to say a word beginning with the facilitating consonant (Dutch method)? Did air enter the esophagus more than once as the patient attempted the model? Once the clinician has determined which behaviors facilitated air loading, stimulus material should be programmed appropriately to reinforce the behavior and to develop the

patient's understanding of what he or she must do to accomplish phonation. It bears repeating that the clinician must obtain many repetitions of the behavior before trying to understand what the patient is
doing when phonation occurs. Again, do not intellectualize the process
too early in therapy. Be sure the behavior is consistent before developing an explicit understanding of the process.

When presenting the model, the clinician may produce the CV stimulus or word using either natural voice, esophageal voice, or glottal fry,
which perceptually resembles esophageal voice. It is not essential that
the clinician be able to use esophageal speech to be successful with laryngectomized patients. Although it may be helpful and is quite easy to
learn, it is not necessary. Our profession calls for us to work with patients
who have cerebral palsy, cleft palates, hearing disorders, stuttering
problems, and so forth, and we do not have to have any of these disorders to be successful.

Direct Approaches

Many laryngectomees will achieve success if the clinician patiently and
repetitiously uses indirect and semidirect approaches. There will always
be those, however, who require a more direct strategy to learn esophageal phonation. Do not make the mistake of prejudging who will or will
not learn via a particular approach. Try to teach all of the methods and
then note what seems, sounds, and looks best for each person. The goal
is to find the easiest and most natural method for each laryngectomized
person.

Direction and clarity of direction is the basic principle in a direct
approach. This is not to say that the use of imagery is precluded in the
direct approach. Imagery can be very helpful for some patients. When
instructing, be sure words do not get in the way. At least initially, avoid
using professional jargon. Simple words should be used to explain the
processes of injection, inhalation, glossopharyngeal press, and so on. The
old adage of "KISS" should always be employed, that is, "Keep it simple,
stupid."

Teaching Air Injection.   My decision to describe separately the techniques to teach injection and those to teach inhalation should not be
interpreted to mean that one method is superior to the other. Nor does
it mean that one is easier to teach than the other. As stated earlier,
many esophageal speakers use a combination of methods, which is
acceptable. The techniques are described separately only to help in
explaining the concepts.

Remember that air injection necessitates closing both the nasal exit
and the oral exit from the mouth and throat. A good beginning is to

show the patient before and after diagrams that appear in the publications by Keith, Shane, Coates, and Devine (1977) and Lauder (1979). Show the patient that the air in the mouth must be forced into the food tube past the closed muscle at the top of that tube and then immediately expelled to vibrate that same muscle. Indicate the continuity of the food tube and stomach and stress the importance of immediately returning any injected air as soon as it is felt to enter the esophagus. The patient must not wait, or the air will be lost to the stomach. Instruct the patient to, "Put some air into your throat and quickly and loudly say /a/." Stay with this approach for several attempts and answer any questions clearly and simply.

If this fails to evoke sound, the clinician who can produce esophageal sound might have the patient touch the clinician's neck during air injection and phonation. The clinician should inject air and phonate several times before asking the patient to try. Be accepting and reassuring of any attempts and do not give up too soon. Make certain that the laryngectomee realizes air must enter the "throat" before sound production can be expected.

If the patient is still unsuccessful, another technique is to have him or her encircle the clinician's neck with his hand and fingers while the clinician alternately tenses and relaxes the neck (pharyngeal) muscles. This results in some pharyngeal constriction and helps to reduce cavity size and hence increase air pressure. Ask the patient to copy the neck tensing and relaxing model. Next, tell the patient to put his or her tongue tip on the gum ridge behind the upper teeth (position for /t/), and to "Push with your tongue while you squeeze your neck muscles." The goal here is to encourage glossal press in addition to some pharyngeal tube contraction. The difficulty the clinician faces with this exercise is having the patient keep the PE segment relaxed while simultaneously tensing pharyngeal and lingual musculature. Clinical ingenuity is needed to create an internal environment that will allow the laryngectomee to utilize these diametrically opposed behaviors. Acceptance, reassurance, and clear verbal prompts in response to what is observed are in order. The patient needs to be relaxed yet also to generate higher intraoral pressure. This is not easy, but it is attainable. If audible air escapes through the mouth, have the patient close the lips while pushing with the tongue. If air escapes through the nose, digitally close the nares.

Next, follow the exact set of instructions just discussed, but this time instruct the patient to place the tip of the tongue on the gum ridge behind the bottom teeth, keep the mouth slightly open, and then move the bulk of the tongue upward and backward. This results in a type of glossopharyngeal press motion. Try both of these tongue maneuvers separately and without the additional pharyngeal (neck muscle) contraction. This may be an important consideration for the patient who evidences a great deal of tension. Also, have the patient try the tongue maneuver with lips open and with lips closed. Some patients may find that with the lips closed an additional pursing and squeezing of the lips further reduces or compresses cavity size and increases the pressure.

Another way to teach injection is to begin by showing the patient that his or her mouth is full of air that can be used for esophageal speech. Light a match, carefully hold it in front of the patient, and ask him or her to blow it out. The odds are that a loud tracheal stoma blast will be heard as the patient futilely tries to blow out the match with pulmonary air. Show him or her that there is more than enough oral air available and how it can be used to blow out a match. The same thing can be demonstrated by using a small whistle, harmonica, oral manometer, straw in a glass of water, strips of paper, and so forth. These activities dramatically show the patient that he or she can indeed build up oral pressure and direct and control air expulsion. Next, ask the patient to close his or her lips and, instead of blowing or squeezing air out through the lips, to squeeze air down into the throat. The patient must use his or her mouth and cheeks like a bellows to force air in the mouth down into the throat and food tube.

Have the patient "push" air into one cheek, into the other cheek (the mouth is kept closed), into the lower lip, into the upper lip, up on the hard palate, back to the soft palate, and finally back on the tonsils and into the throat. Contracting the muscles in the neck and throat (as previously described) during this exercise may provide some additional help in increasing pressure to inject the air.

Also try using language to develop concepts that offer a target for charging the esophagus with air. The direction to "pump air into your throat," "shovel air into your throat," "scoop some air into your throat," "squeeze," "compress," "push," "force," "shove," "gargle," and so forth, may evoke the desired behavior. Try to find a word that offers an appropriate image for each person. I remember one man for whom the command, "Use your tongue like a piston to drive the air in," worked beautifully. The man happened to be a mechanic. It was a good thing that the command alone worked, because I must confess that I do not even know what a piston is. For additional ideas regarding imagery to evoke esophageal sound, see the works by Salmon (1971) and Shanks and Duguay (1984).

Teaching Air Inhalation.   A technique I have found to be very successful for teaching inhalation is to ask the patient to relax and to yawn as deeply, easily, and realistically as possible. If the clinician listens carefully, he or she will often hear a faint click or popping sound at the height of a "good" yawn. This is the PE segment opening as oropharyngeal air is drawn into the esophagus because of increased negative esophageal pressure associated with exaggerated inspiratory movement accompanying the yawn. If the sound is heard, identify it and reinforce more productions. Next, ask the patient to produce sound as the air is forced out of the esophagus. Help the patient maintain quiet, comfortable, and relaxed sound production because tension from increased effort may serve to tighten the PE segment. Move from the sound (usually a neutral, schwa-like sound) on exhalation to other close vowels and then to VC combinations ("up," "out," "at," "on," "off," etc.). Work to habituate the behavior.

Another technique requires the clinician to manually cover his or her nose and mouth to demonstrate that breathing can be stopped for a few seconds without danger of suffocation. In turn, the laryngectomee is instructed to hold his or her breath by covering the stoma with the finger(s). Have the patient do this for a few brief seconds, and then to remove his or her hand and breathe. Repeat this a few times until the patient understands that he or she will not suffocate if the stoma is covered for a moment. Next, instruct the patient to exhale completely and then occlude the tracheostoma with his or her finger(s). The patient should then open the mouth and quickly and vigorously suck air into the mouth and throat. If this three-part maneuver (exhale–cover–suck in) is successful, sound will occur as the air is "inhaled" through the PE segment and into the esophagus. This technique may also be tried without covering the stoma. However, the thoracic cavity should be held somewhat fixed to minimize the accompanying pulmonary inhalation. Care should be taken to ensure that the patient, although working hard, is relaxed since tension in the PE segment must be overcome upon inhalation. If sound occurs it should be identified, reinforced, and then "reversed" so that it occurs on exhalation. The sound of the air entering the esophagus will then need to be extinguished. It is not uncommon to hear a patient who is just learning this technique start to speak on inhalation. Obviously, this must be reversed since the esophagus is the reservoir for the air used in esophageal speech.

Another way to teach inhalation is through imagery. Such words as "sniff air in," "draw air into your throat," "suck air into your mouth and throat," and "pretend you are gargling glass," can prove helpful. Again, the reader is encouraged to examine the works of Salmon (1971) and Shanks and Duguay (1984) for a more complete discussion of the use of imagery in esophageal speech therapy.

Air Expulsion—If a Problem. The expulsion of esophageal air is a complex process. Just as focusing on how injection or inhalation occurs can interfere with the naturalness of the process, so can focusing on air expulsion. Throughout this chapter the emphasis has been on eliciting the behavior, eliciting the behavior again, repeating the behavior, repeating the behavior again, and only then determining what accounts for the behavior. Do not focus on air expulsion unless it becomes a problem. It should be a natural and easy process for the patient to return the injected/inhaled air. If, however, the patient has never produced any esophageal phonation (with the exception of spontaneous eructations), and the clinician "knows" that air has entered the esophagus, then air expulsion must be addressed.

Sometimes a patient does a good job of getting air in, but then simply opens his or her mouth and expects the "speech fairy" to talk for him or her. The patient does not realize that he or she must actively participate to drive the air (sound) back out. To involve the patient in air expulsion, first help identify the exact moment that air enters the esophagus. Do this with tactile cues (put his or her hand and fingers to the neck in the area of the PE segment) and, if necessary, with auditory cues (amplification). Sometimes it is even possible to identify air intake visually. There may be a slight bulging out of neck tissue in the region of the PE segment that can be seen as well as palpated. When the patient has an understanding of air entering, say, "Just as soon as you feel or hear the air enter, as loud as you can, say /a/." (Also try "uh," "up," or some other VC combination.) Try some front, mid, or back vowel singletons or VC combinations to vary the tension of the musculature. In some instances, simply making sounds instead of producing meaningful utterances may be better practice because the communication element may supersede the motor performance, generate tension, and result in failure. Emphasize the need to say it loudly, stoma blasts and all. When one speaks loudly there is an accompanying increase in expiration effort. One employs active rather than passive expiratory behavior. The muscles of expiration function mechanically to (a) lower the ribs and/or sternum; (b) decrease the anterior, posterior, and transverse dimensions of the thorax; (c) raise abdominal pressures forcing the diaphragm upward; and (d) decrease the vertical dimension of the thorax. Loud talking increases this maneuver, which helps to collapse the esophagus, thus assisting in driving the air back out.

If asking the patient to talk louder does not accomplish the goal of driving air/sound back out, help the patient with timing of air expulsion. The most important muscles for active expiration, sometimes referred to collectively as the abdominal muscles, include the rectus abdominus, external oblique, and transverse abdominus. They function to draw the lower ribs and sternum downward, force the abdominal contents inward, and raise abdominal pressure. Assisting in active respiration are 11 thin muscles situated within the rib interspaces underneath the external intercostals. They are collectively referred to as the internal intercostals. Upon contraction, they pull the ribs downward and stiffen the rib interspaces. Most of this action can be felt and/or seen. To help the patient with timing of air expulsion, the clinician's hand is placed on the area medial and just inferior to the thoracic (rib) cage. The patient is asked to consciously practice alternately tensing and relaxing those muscles. Watch that he or she does not thrust the abdomen out. The patient is to tighten the muscles, not belly dance. To help further identify the area that needs to be tensed, have the patient "pant" while showing him or her the area. Once this tensing ability has been established and is under good volitional control, add the instruction, "Pretend to say /a/ when I push on the spot and you tighten." The patient is to pretend saying /a/ and tightening until good muscle contraction occurs in immediate response to the "fingers push" stimulus. Finally, have the patient load air; just as soon as it is heard entering the esophagus, push and have him or her say /a/. Do not let the patient quit the attempt to phonate too soon. Make sure he or she keeps on tensing so that perhaps some of the air can be forced up before it gets into the lower esophagus and/or stomach. Drill on this for some time until the fingers push stimulus can gradually be faded.

Another way to assist training in air expulsion is to have the patient load air and then quickly pull up on something heavy (a radiator, window ledge, etc.), and phonate. As before, have the patient maintain that tension for a while in order to return at least some of the air charge.

In The Event of No Sound

The clinician must create a relaxed and comfortable therapy environment. Tension has to be reduced since it can negatively affect PE segment function. The physical environment, as well as the clinician's comfort level, ease, reassurance, and sense of humor, all work to create the optimum condition for the initiation of phonation. The clinician should not rush through all the techniques that have been suggested. Proceed very slowly, easily, and for some time with each technique. Build a solid foundation upon which to develop the next level. If, however, the clinician has honestly and patiently tried all of the techniques described here and in other sources, and still has never heard any sound of air entering the esophagus, this may be a "no win" situation. The most obvious barrier to air intake procedures is a PE segment in tonic resistance. The recommendation is to perform an air insufflation test as described in chapter 6.

DEVELOPING SPEECH

Once esophageal sound has been established, the next step is to develop consistency of phonation. In behavioral terms, the patient needs to develop the ability to reliably, consistently, and at will phonate 9 of 10 consecutive VC or CV syllables on 10 separate air charges, with little or no effort and with a latency of 0.5 s or less between separate sounds (Berlin, 1963). The other latency measure that is critical is the time between air in and sound out, which must be in the neighborhood of 0.4 to 0.2 s (Shanks, 1986). Some laryngectomees want to talk so badly that they often end up just that way—talking so badly. Practice does not make perfect. One gets what one practices, and only perfect practice makes perfect. When the new laryngectomee realizes that he or she can make sound and say words, he or she uses the only developing ability to communicate. As a result, the patient practices and reinforces undesirable and bad habits. The amount of time spent each day communicating versus the time spent practicing good speech skills is vastly uneven. The new laryngectomee should be strongly encouraged to use an artificial device for the bulk of his or her communication needs and then to practice esophageal speech as perfectly as possible, frequently and for short periods of time. Staggered practice is superior to a long, intensive practice session. I often suggest practice during television commercials. They are short but frequent.

The next step in therapy, which will occupy the majority of training from this point on, is to develop adequate length of phonation. The patient must train his or her new phonatory mechanism to produce esophageal sound for a sufficient duration of time to allow him or her to say complete phrases and sentences. It is helpful clinically to chart this temporal behavior as a visual record of progress. Chart two behaviors: the number of vowel sounds per air charge, and the length of vowel phonation. The reason for charting vowels is to prevent duration measurements from being contaminated by any gains that may be attributed to consonant injection. If the patient happens to be a consonant injector and still needs to employ the consonant in order to take in air, merely have him or her say, "tah ah ah ah ah" and "taaa . . . h" for these two vowel measures. When these measures are recorded for all vowels and diphthongs, a rather linear progression of the skill will be noted as proficiency develops. This will not change appreciably from session to session, but rather is a gradual skill acquisition with plateaus along the way. The patient's goal is production of eight, nine, or more vowels per air charge and a phonation duration of 2 s or more. This phonatory length is sufficient for most of the demands of our language. This, of course, assumes that the other dimensions of speaking such as intelligibility, loudness, stress, and so forth, are also acquired. Duration can be developed by "stretching out" vowels, diphthongs, monosyllabic words, and selected polysyllabic words ("around," "almond," "animal," etc.) that do not phonetically permit "sneaking in" air from loading consonant sounds. If the patient still needs the consonant to load air, the drills could use the loading consonant followed by a vowel or vowels, or such word combinations as "tie it," "tie up," or even "tie ah ah."

This might be a good place in therapy to start to "wean" the consonant injector from consonant dependency. The author remembers with great love and affection a past president of the International Association of Laryngectomees (IAL), a consonant injector who always referred to the organization as the "KI KA KL." Of course, it is the motor movement, rather than the consonant per se, that accounts for the injection of air. If, for example, the goal is to extinguish the consonant T as a loader, ask the patient to say the word "eye." Because it is a diphthong, he will be unable to say the word. Then have him repeat the word "tie" several times. Tell him, "Start to say the word 'tie,' but at the last second, just as soon as you feel the air go in, say 'eye.' " Do this several times; then tell him, "Make a silent /t/ and say 'tie.' " Do this same thing for the following stimuli: "ape," "all," "air," "ale," and "ache." Finally, switch to words such as "up," "on," "itch," and "yes." This same protocol can be used to fade the consonant dependency but keep the needed motor movement for those patients who use /k/, /p/, /t/, and so forth, to initiate injection.

As drills to develop length of phonation proceed, try using a carrier phrase of four words followed by two more words. For example, use "I saw a big" followed by "red car," "fat man," "old tree," "new plane," and so forth. Then the patient is instructed to "phrase" the sentence into two, three, four, five, and six words per air charge, for example, "I saw – a big – red car," "I saw a – big red car," "I saw a big – red car," "I saw a big red – car," and finally "I saw a big red car." The use of poems, newspapers, and materials from the patient's work or recreational environment can be used as material for drill on length of phonation. Clinical skills come into play to find varied and interesting ways to develop length of phonation—a skill critical to esophageal speech proficiency.

ADDITIONAL CONSIDERATIONS

Articulation

The single most important factor that contributes to intelligibility of esophageal speech is articulation. The patient often is a middle-aged or older person who may present with presbycusis. Be certain to evaluate hearing status and to focus on any related articulation errors. Carefully listen for any consonant sound confusions and omissions of final consonant sounds in the patient's speech. Also, as discussed earlier, be sure that he or she does not intrude the sound of a loading consonant in words. The clinician's training in conventional articulation therapy will provide the management skills necessary to handle these problems.

A couple of additional errors are inherent to esophageal speech. One is with the nasals /m/, /n/, and /ŋ/. During injection (and often even during inhalation), the nasal port is closed off (i.e., velopharyngeal valving). Some patients may forget to drop the velum or may accomplish this too slowly, resulting in loss of nasality for the normally nasalized consonants. Having the patient practice humming overcomes this closure problem and creates an awareness of both the sound and feel of nasalization. The awareness of nasalization can be transferred to words beginning and ending with nasals through drill activities designed for this purpose.

The other major articulatory problem is with the /h/ sound. Because it is a glottal aspirate, it cannot be articulated after laryngectomy. Several communication strategies can be employed, however, to increase /h/ word intelligibility. Encourage the patient to use the troublesome /h/ word in a sentence or phrase, preferably a sentence. The increased length of the message unit, with all of the additional clues it provides, almost guarantees recognition of the /h/ sound.

Another therapy technique takes advantage of the temporal dimension of the /h/ sound. It takes longer to say "hat" than to say "at." Therefore, have the patient prolong the initial vowel sound in the word (/æ/ in hat) so that temporally the listener "hears" or furnishes the missing /h/ that "seems" to be present. Drills can be devised to practice this skill using word contrasts such as "at–hat," "ate–hate," "ale–hale," "owe–hoe," and so forth.

This type of pairing also can be used if there is listener confusion with an /h/ word. Have the patient deliberately say the misperceived word followed by the prolonged intended word. "I didn't say 'and', I said 'aaand' " (i.e., "hand").

A stomal /h/ is difficult to master and is almost impossible to use in rapid conversational speech; yet, the stomal /h/ can be extremely effective for particular speech needs. The patient simply makes an audible stomal exhalation and then voices the remainder of the word (e.g., "Pay attention, I said *H*ackett"). This is especially useful for individuals who have last names beginning with the /h/ sound where the technique of embedding the word in a larger message unit would be of little value. Generally, patients find this practice fun.

Distracting Behaviors

Speech needs to both sound good and look good. Several common unde-sireable habits can work against that end. They need to be identified early and immediately extinguished before they become practiced esophageal speech behavior.

Stoma Blasts. Stoma blasts occur frequently and are difficult to reverse. They result from the turbulent flow of air through the tracheal tube. The blast is the forceful and quick expulsion of pulmonary air. The patient needs to slow down the airflow by expelling it more slowly. The first order of business is to help the patient become aware of this stoma noise. The presence of presbycusis in this population is signifi-cant and adds to the difficulty of the patient's hearing stoma noise. The use of amplifying equipment with the microphone held directly over the stoma may help to heighten the patient's perception. Also, holding a small piece of paper in front of the stoma during phonation can provide visual evidence. Especially helpful devices to use for awareness are the stethoscope or a set of earphones such as those used to listen to music on commercial airline flights. The ear pieces are placed in the patient's ears, and the other end is held over the stoma during phonation. This method often results in the patient's dramatic realization of the problem. If he or she cannot "internally" make the necessary adjustment to eliminate the stomal noise, telling the patient to "slow down the flow" and "let it out easily" may help.

One should also carefully determine whether there is a particular place in an utterance where the blast becomes more noticeable. It is not uncommon to hear the blast at the end of a phrase or sentence when the patient is forcing very hard to get out the last few words. The increased effort results in increased airflow speed and, hence, stoma noise. The patient is instructed to say, and to practice, fewer words per air charge until longer sound duration free of stoma noise is developed and available for speech.

Stoma blasts also result from the increased effort demanded for loud talking. Reduce the intensity level to reduce the effort, thereby reduc-ing the airflow speed and noise. It is important to work toward over-coming the dual problems of hearing loss in the older patient and the auditory feedback system intensity level that he or she has habituated over decades of life. The patient, who is used to speaking at a certain intensity level, still aims for this acoustic target after laryngectomy, in spite of the fact that it can never be achieved in esophageal speech. The esophageal speaker utilizes an intensity level that averages 6–10 dB less than normal speech (Robbins, Fisher, Blom, & Singer, 1984). He or she must be helped to adjust to a reduced phonatory intensity. Speaking more clearly, not loudly, is the goal.

Because the problem is an acoustic one, the hearing status of the patient should be carefully assessed and appropriate measures taken. Amplification may be needed for the patient and, just as importantly, for the spouse if he or she has a hearing loss that requires the laryngectomee to talk louder in order to be heard. Examine the speaking environment at home and at work, and help make any necessary adjustments and corrections. Stoma noise is a real problem and one that requires vigorous and persistent attention to minimize and control.

Air Klunking. Another common and persistent distracting behavior is the audible klunking sound of the air charge entering the esophagus. Experience suggests that this problem is more common in the patient who injects air than in the one who uses an inhalation technique. As with stoma noise, the patient must first be made aware of this behavior. Amplifying devices can be used to heighten the sound of the klunk. Tactile feedback also can be provided by having the laryngectomee hold his or her hand to the neck with the fingers over the approximate site of the PE segment. Once the patient realizes what he or she is doing, work can commence to eliminate or minimize the klunk.

Because klunking is more common among injecters, try switching these patients to an inhalation method of air intake. This is not always possible because a patient may be unable to sufficiently relax the PE segment for inhalation and may need to use injection techniques to increase oropharyngeal pressure, thereby overriding the tonic resistance of the barrier. Nevertheless, first try to switch to an inhalation technique.

The next step is to try to vary the method of injection. The general belief (e.g., Diedrich & Youngstrom, 1966) is that klunking results from too much air being used too quickly and with too great an effort. For this reason, try consonant injection to reduce the klunk. The use of a consonant encourages less air intake, requires less effort and tension buildup, and helps "mask" the klunk somewhat since the klunk is partially obscured by the sounds preceding and following it in a word.

The type of injection might also be varied in an effort to minimize the sound. Have a patient who uses lip injection switch to tongue injection. Less successful, but sometimes helpful, is to move the tongue injector to lip injection. Also, try injecting with the tongue tip up and then the tip down to see if any improvement results.

Listen very carefully to a sample of conversational speech and record that sample. Determine whether there were any occurrences of air intake with little or no klunking. If so, identify these occurrences, reinforce them, and drill to create the desired pattern of loading air.

Klunking and stoma noises are perhaps the two most common and annoying behaviors employed by laryngectomized speakers. The behaviors are easily developed and reinforced and, for this reason, should not be "practiced" in early communication. The artificial larynx can be used for lengthy communication early in therapy. Careful monitoring and follow-up need to be continued so that the patient does not lapse into the behaviors again once they are corrected or minimized. One should also keep in mind the value of negative practice as an important clinical technique to address the problem of klunking and/or stoma noise.

Visual Distractors. The good esophageal speaker, like the laryngeal speaker, is considerate of his listener. Both want the message, not the way they say the message, to be of primary importance. For this reason, the clinician must help the patient identify and remediate any visual mannerisms that detract and distract from oral communication. The patient may have acquired and reinforced facial grimaces, lip smacking, double loading behavior, extraneous head and shoulder movements, poor eye contact, and so forth, as negative accompaniment to air trapping. A former student of mine once referred to these unnecessary movements as "secondaries" in the same sense as those mannerisms adopted by stutterers. Sometimes the listener even tells the laryngectomized speaker to, "Take it easy" or "Don't try so hard to talk." In short, by employing these secondary behaviors, the speaker gives the visual impression that he or she finds it very difficult and demanding to talk. These problems can be approached in the same manner one approaches extinguishing secondary behaviors in stutterers. Mirror work and videotaping can be used for identification; then cancellations, negative practice, and so on, can be used with excellent results.

Quality of Voice. Like mercy, the quality of esophageal speech should not be strained. It also should be as pleasant and as normal as possible. Achieving normal quality in esophageal speech is not easy because the fundamental frequency of esophageal speech is significantly lower than that of normal speech. There is, however, a wide range of individual differences exhibited by speakers. Weinberg and Bennett (1972) reported a range from 34 to 83 Hz for their male subjects and from 33 to 200 Hz for their female subjects. The average fundamental frequency is 58 Hz for males and 87 Hz for females. This is consistent with the notion that the fundamental frequency for male esophageal speakers is about an octave lower than that of the adult male laryngeal speaker.

In addition to the lower fundamental frequency, the perception of esophageal speech as being monotonous lies in part with the listener's difficulty in discriminating subtle low-frequency differences. Fortunately, however, the excellent esophageal speaker has available a fairly substantial pitch range (Damsté, 1958; Hoops & Noll, 1969; Kytta, 1964; Shipp, 1967; Snidecor, 1940; Snidecor & Curry, 1959; Tato, Mariani,

DePicolli, & Mirasov, 1954). Lessons and drills should be devised to capitalize and expand upon the patient's pitch range. Singing with an esophageal voice can create a dramatic awareness of pitch changing ability. The use of songs that are both familiar and simple can be incorporated into therapy at both individual and group levels. To help the patient approximate more normal phonation, the clinician should try to develop and reinforce use of the upper, higher part of the patient's esophageal voice range.

In addition to the singing and humming drills, conventional speech exercises for expanding the vocal range of other voice patients can be used. These include drills with the "wh" words, interrogative sentences, poetry, and role playing.

Refinement of esophageal speech is generally neglected. Frequently, when a patient develops serviceable esophageal voice, he or she terminates therapy. In fairness to both patient and clinician, the termination of therapy often is influenced by financial considerations and/or travel constraints. It would be beneficial if the clinician could invest as much time as needed to refine and polish the esophageal voice of an alaryngeal speaker who is willing and motivated to achieve excellence. Clinicians need to motivate and challenge the laryngectomized patient to achieve excellence. Clinicians must employ the readily available videotape recorder to allow patients to both see and hear their communication efforts so that they can join in identifying behaviors that can be improved or irradicated. Hopefully, one day a serviceable esophageal voice will not be considered enough, but rather excellence of esophageal speech will be the standard.

Beatitudes of a Laryngectomized Person

Blessed are you who take the time
    to listen to my strange new speech.
    For you help me to realize
    that I can be understood.
Blessed are you who never ask me to "hurry up"
    or say my words for me.
    For I appreciate the time extended—
    more than help intended.
Blessed are you who do not shout at me
    when I speak.
    For you realize that I am not deaf . . .
    only sometimes a little dumb.
Blessed are you who ask me to repeat
    when you do not understand me.
    For that is more honest and helpful
    than pretending you understand.

Blessed are you who allow me
    new opportunities and challenges to use my speech.
    For only by doing and succeeding
    will I grow in confidence and ability.
Blessed are my doctors, nurses, my speech clinician,
    all my friends and especially my family.
    For you have given me back my life
    and helped me realize how very fortunate and lucky I am.
Blessed are you who love me
    just as I am.

REFERENCES

Atkinson, M., Kramer, P., Wyman, S. M., & Inglefinger, F. J. (1957). The dynamics of swallowing: I. Normal pharyngeal mechanisms. *Journal of Clinical Investigation, 36,* 581–588.

Berlin, C. I. (1963). Clinical measurement of esophageal speech: I. Methodology and curves of skill acquisition. *Journal of Speech and Hearing Disorders, 28,* 42–51.

Damsté, P. H. (1958). *Oesophageal speech.* Groningen, The Netherlands: Gebroeders Hoitsema.

Decroix, G., Libersa, C., & Lattard, R. (1958). Bases anstomiques et physiologiques de la reeducation vocale des laryngectomisés [The anatomical and physiological foundations of voice reeducation in laryngectomees]. *Journal of Français d' Otolaryngologie, 7,* 549–573.

Dey, F. L., & Kirchner, J. A. (1961). The upper esophageal sphincter after laryngectomy. *Laryngoscope, 71,* 99–115.

DiCarlo, L., Amster, W., & Herer, G. (1956). *Speech after laryngectomy.* Syracuse, NY: Syracuse University Press.

Diedrich, W. M., & Youngstrom, K. A. (1966). *Alaryngeal speech.* Springfield, IL: Charles C. Thomas.

Duguay, M. J. (1968). In E. Lauder, The laryngectomee and the artificial larynx. *Journal of Speech and Hearing Disorders, 33,* 147–157.

Duguay, M. J. (1978). Why not both? In S. J. Salmon & L. P. Goldstein (Eds.), *The artificial larynx handbook* (pp. 3–10). New York: Grune and Stratton.

Duguay, M. J. (1986). Using speech aid(e)s. In J. C. Shanks (Ed.), Current strategies of rehabilitation of the laryngectomized patient, in W. H. Perkins & J. L. Northern (Eds.), *Seminars in Speech and Language, 7*(1), 13–29. New York: Thieme.

Hodson, C. J., & Oswald, M. V. D. (1958). *Speech recovery after total laryngectomy.* Baltimore: Williams & Wilkins.

Hoops, H. R., & Noll, J. D. (1969). Relationship of selected acoustic variables to judgments of esophageal speech. *Journal of Communication Disorders, 2,* 1–13.

Keith, R. L., Shane, H. C., Coates, M. B., & Devine, K. D. (1977). *Looking forward: A guidebook for the laryngectomee.* Rochester, NY: Mayo Foundation.

Kytta, J. (1964). Spectographic studies of the sound quality of oesophageal speech. *Acta Oto-Laryngology Supplement, 188,* 371–378.

Lauder, E. (1979). *Self help for laryngectomee.* San Antonio, TX: Author.

Moolenaar-Bijl, A. (1953a). Connection between consonant articulation and the intake of air in esophageal speech. *Folia Phoniatrica, 5,* 212–215.

Moolenaar-Bijl, A. (1953b). The importance of certain consonants in esophageal voice after laryngectomy. *Annals of Otology, Rhinology and Laryngology, 62,* 979–989.

Motta, G., Profazio, A., & Acciarri, T. (1959). Roentgenocinematographic observations on the phonation of laryngectomized subjects. *Otorhinolaring (Ital), 28,* 261–286.

Robbins, J., Fisher, H. B., Blom, E. D., & Singer, M. I. (1984). A comparative acoustic study of normal, esophageal, and tracheoesophageal speech production. *Journal of Speech and Hearing Disorders, 49,* 202–210.

Robe, E. Y., Moore, P., Andrews, A. H., Jr., & Holinger, P. H. (1956). A study of the role of certain factors in the development of speech with respiration. *Laryngoscope, 66,* 173–186 (Part 1), 382–401 (Part 2), 418–499 (Part 3).

Salmon, S. J. (1971). Use of imagery in teaching esophageal speech. *California Journal of Communication Disorders, 2,* 17–24.

Schlosshauer, B., & Mockel, G. (1958). Interpretation of roentgen sound film made of esophageal speakers. *Folia Phoniatrica, 10,* 154–166.

Shanks, J. C. (1986). Developing esophageal communication. In R. L. Keith & F. L. Darley (Eds.), *Laryngectomee rehabilitation* (2nd ed., pp. 71–83). Austin, TX: PRO-ED.

Shanks, J. C., & Duguay, M. J. (1984). Voice remediation and the teaching of alaryngeal speech. In S. Dickson (Ed.), *Communication disorder: Remedial principles and practices* (pp. 240–287). Chicago: Scott Foresman.

Shipp, T. (1967). Frequency, duration, and perceptual measures in relation to judgments of alaryngeal speech acceptability. *Journal of Speech and Hearing Research, 10,* 417–427.

Snidecor, J. (1940). *Experimental studies of the pitch and duration characteristics of superior speech.* Unpublished doctoral dissertation, State University of Iowa, Iowa City.

Snidecor, J., & Curry, E. T. (1959). Temporal and pitch aspects of superior esophageal speech. *Annals of Otology, Rhinology and Laryngology, 68,* 623–636.

Snidecor, J. C., & Isshiki, N. (1965). Air volume and air flow relationships of six male esophageal speakers. *Journal of Speech and Hearing Disorders, 30,* 205–215.

Tato, J. M., Mariani, N., DePicolli, E., & Mirasov, P. (1954). Study of the sonospectrographic characteristics of the voice in laryngectomized patients. *Acta Otolaryngology, 44,* 431–438.

Vrticka, K., & Svoboda, M. (1961). A clinical and x-ray study of 100 laryngectomized speakers. *Folia Phoniatrica, 13,* 174–186.

Weinberg, B., & Bennett, S. (1972). Selected acoustic characteristics of esophageal speech produced by female laryngectomees. *Journal of Speech and Hearing Research, 15,* 211–216.

CHAPTER 4

Toward Advancing Esophageal Communication

Samuel K. Haroldson

Haroldson asserts that in an ongoing clinical program the roles of client and clinician eventually become reversed. His premise is that the clinician must help the client assume an active role in identifying and modifying undesirable behaviors. Haroldson's unusual clinical approach enables clients to gain insights about their behaviors so that their motivation to change is self-generated.

Study Questions

1. What are the implications of differentiating between speech and voice in planning a program of treatment for the laryngectomee?
2. How can group process be utilized in the ongoing development of esophageal voice?
3. Why involve the spouse or significant others in the specifics of an esophageal voice program?

A number of biases are implied with the words used to title this chapter. The word *toward* means movement to a direction and does not necessarily mean a goal. This is not to say that goals are not important, but rather to suggest that improving esophageal communication may well become a way of life. The word *advancing* relates more to the individual's attainment of maximum potential rather than how the individual's performance compares with others. Although the *esophageal* speaker is the primary focus of the discussion, I do not mean to imply in any way that speakers using alternative forms of alaryngeal voicing are less advanced or desirable. Finally, the word *communication* is chosen to convey the ongoing process in the broadest possible sense. Too often, terms like esophageal become attached to speech, resulting in a misnomer. In many instances, speech is intact and it is the alaryngeal voice we are striving to develop and perfect. We are well aware of the uniqueness of human communication and the fact that this separates us from other life forms that use nonhuman communication. Bryngelson (1966) liked to refer to humans as "talking primates," stressing their uniqueness and the importance of what comes out of their mouths. Verbal communication is a process used by humans to share with each other, and it is this process that clinicians are seeking to refine or restore with esophageal speakers.

Many aspects of the communication process seem relevant. Clients and their listeners are surprised to realize how much of their communication involves lipreading. By covering our mouths and/or faces, we can easily demonstrate our dependencies on visual cues. Within this same context, people often realize they are quite adept at lipreading. Focusing upon and experimenting with visual cues result in positive changes for many laryngectomees and their listeners.

Another aspect of the communication process that is unfamiliar to many clients and their families is the differentiation of speech, voice, and language. The distinguishing characteristics can be illustrated by encouraging people to look at what is being said versus how it is being said. One of the most comforting accomplishments is when laryngectomees move beyond saying, "I had my voice box removed and now I can't talk." Understanding and appreciating the differences between speech and voice are necessary for patients and professionals because such awareness is basic to the rehabilitation process.

Another aspect of the communication process worthy of explanation is the fact that vocabularies (including expletives) have not disappeared as a result of laryngectomy. Many mental, emotional, and social characteristics of our personalities are manifested in the language we use, and surgery does not alter this fact.

THE ONGOING REFINEMENT PROGRAM

Under this very broad heading, we are concerned about the client's own program for living with and communicating with an esophageal voice. Because a refinement program is the topic, the underlying assumption is that the speaker has learned to produce esophageal voice consistently and is capable of functional communication. Another assumption is that this individual is a successful artificial larynx user.

We are interested in describing an ongoing refinement program, a program whereby the clients are learning to be their own clinicians, thereby learning to evaluate and modify their own behavior. Such a program will help clients to develop their own communication process. They must acquire a certain level of patience and acceptance, yet retain enough curiosity to be sufficiently challenged to attempt continued change.

Within this program, clients must learn to define and establish their own goals. Developing a goal that becomes a constant across a variety of speaking situations is often beneficial. The goal remains the same, but the complexity and difficulty of the situations are varied. Clients should not confuse their goals with the techniques used to meet them. For example, while reporting about the goal to monitor and modify stomal activity across various levels of situational difficulty, a client may reveal confusion about the differences between the goal and how to attempt to implement (practice) the goal. Defining a single goal and working systematically toward the implementation of that goal can do a great deal to simplify the process of positive change.

In 1957, Williams described some therapeutic techniques for stuttering which over time have proven relevant to a variety of clinical areas. Williams emphasized the importance of defining a goal positively in terms of what we are asking the client to do rather than not do. If we apply this concept to an esophageal speaker who exhibits stomal noise or blowing, we might ask the client to focus on easy expulsion of air rather than asking him or her not to blow or to stop blowing. Although the difference between these approaches may seem inconsequential, it is encouraging to observe clients alter their behavior when they become involved in this process of positively approaching change.

Another component of the program involves teaching and encouraging the client to evaluate carefully his or her own behavior. Duguay (1986) described the process very well in terms of practice, evaluate, and proceed to practice again. The temporal relationship between the practice effort and the client's evaluation of his or her performance should be as immediate as possible so that the effectiveness of the evaluation is maximized.

This is the time to underscore the advantage of functioning in the here and now. Essentially, it is impossible to change behavior any time other than now. Assisting a patient in learning to reduce worry and concern about the past or future can help in profound ways, not only at the level of voice production, but possibly in many other facets of life. This kind of clinical direction can make an individual's program more fulfilling and rewarding.

Currently, a preponderance of programs exist that emphasize 12 steps that focus on overcoming and accepting a number of very human conditions. Perhaps the largest and oldest is Alcoholics Anonymous. Acceptance, honesty, and gratitude are but a few of the obvious tenets encouraged in these programs, but which apply to all humans. Clinicians might find it helpful to familiarize themselves with the tenets of these programs (see, e.g., Mendelson & Mello, 1985; Robertson, 1988). In some instances, clinical practice may become more effective by using a similar holistic approach.

A very natural bond often exists between the principles of a 12-step program and the processes we have been discussing regarding the habituation and refinement of a new voice. For example, one of the basic principles of 12-step programs is acceptance. Laryngectomees might apply this principle to themselves and strive for acceptance of the disease, cancer, or acceptance of changes (and limitations) in their voices. For some, this process generates the ability to evaluate honestly personal potential for change. To consider one's limitations and learn to solicit honest feedback from others becomes an interesting process. Obviously, the programs being discussed focus on activities highly dependent upon talking and listening. While engaging in these activities, laryngectomized speakers obtain esophageal voice practice, as well as an opportunity to address a variety of personal needs. Through the years, more than one client has been "referred" (nudged) into various treatment programs under the guise of providing a good opportunity to practice speaking. Some very interesting changes (including voice) have evolved.

Specific Areas of Refinement

The word *refinement* implies that we are focusing on the honing and polishing aspect of esophageal speech. I have long felt that the refinement of esophageal speech can best be implemented in a format that includes individual contact with the professional and a substantial amount of group interaction. Group interaction is defined as a gathering of two or more clients.

The group process lends itself to accomplishments in many areas. Feedback and interaction among laryngectomees are often unique and provide a potent vehicle for clinical change. A concept or point of view exchanged between laryngectomees may have much more effect than the same information exchanged between a laryngectomee and professional. Obviously, on occasion the converse might be true. When the group process is acting effectively, the clinician can contribute most by knowing when to stay out of the way and being capable of doing so.

Speech Production and Modification. Speech patterns and habits are well established and are changed very slowly over time, if at all. As one client reminded the group, "habit is a cable. We weave a thread of it every day until at last it becomes so strong we cannot break it." Fortunately, the potential for changing habits is not quite so bleak as the client suggested, or many professionals would have left the field in pursuit of greener pastures. However, for most clients, this process of behavioral change requires changing patterns that have become highly habituated over lifetimes of 40, 50, 60, or more years. It is little wonder that change takes time. Viewing change from this perspective is often comforting to the client who has plateaued or become discouraged with a seeming lack of progress.

Rate is considered an important aspect of speaking and has been a topic of almost universal clinical discussion and concern. What is an appropriate rate of speech, and by what standards is it determined? Like many stutterers, laryngectomees frequently report the almost hewn cry of listeners, "Slow down, you're talking too fast. Take your time." Such reports are frequently made by clients when they begin communicating with an electrolarynx. And why should clinicians be surprised? After all, the laryngectomees are using lifelong patterns that were not at all affected by the amputation of their larynges. Why should laryngectomees not attempt to utilize the same rate they have used all their lives?

When the subject of changing rate is discussed with a client, the nearly universal instruction involves some variation of "slow down." When we pursue the effectiveness of this instruction, however, it becomes obvious that such a directive is a fairly impractical, unmanageable goal to keep in mind over time. Clients report great difficulty in consciously maintaining a slow pace. Frequently, a rapid speaking rate is only one part of a larger pattern of behavior. Rapid talkers often think, eat, walk, and drive rapidly, as well. For them, speaking rapidly literally has become a way of life. It is understandable how the overused clinical phrase "Take time to talk" evolved and why it is a most meaningful goal when attempting to change rate as well as other facets of esophageal communication.

Many clinicians agree that success of the communication process can best be determined by ascertaining the listener's ability to understand the message. Accordingly, clinicians are interested in "stacking the deck" in favor of the listener's understanding. This concept coincides nicely with the concept of taking time to talk (i.e., changing speaking rate). There is nothing quite like encouragement from the listener who says, "Hey, I can understand you so much better when you take your time."

Some clinicians develop the skill of demonstrating how a rapid rate affects such aspects as articulation, intelligibility, and even listener's attention. In some cases, building a clinical library of audio and video samples can be very helpful in teaching a client to define and evaluate accurate attainable goals. A group setting can provide a valuable arena for practice. Also, efforts made to use appropriate rate while speaking with an artificial larynx will reduce the usual therapy time required to achieve appropriate rate for esophageal speech.

Finally, the physical and mechanical constraints involved in producing esophageal voice may be the most salient factors that convince the client to reduce rate. The voicing mechanism will not operate with the same speed as it did presurgically.

| *Articulation.* | A direct relationship exists between articulation and esophageal voice production. In an excellent chapter entitled "Evoking Esophageal Voice," Shanks (1986) described this relationship in a functional, straightforward manner. Shanks emphasized the importance of articulatory precision and of explaining that the tendency of some esophageal speakers to tighten or tense the tongue and lips during esophageal insufflation may have an adverse effect on their articulation. Shanks also indicated that as esophageal phonation improves and becomes more automatic, some speakers demonstrate a concomitant change in speaking proficiency.

Another important aspect in working on articulation involves experimenting with the size of the oral cavity. Enlarging the resonating cavity by dropping the jaw often improves the intelligibility and intensity of the esophageal voice. Experimentation of this type often results in immediate changes that can be dramatic, surprising, and often exciting. Again, the group setting provides a source for reinforcement and a more lifelike environment for experimentation and practice.

Evaluating change over time can be difficult for clinicians. One interesting measure of longitudinal change is the emergence of the speaker's foreign or regional dialect. One client, a native of Ireland, began to make great clinical strides when several members of the group commented on his Irish brogue. This appeared to be a pivotal point in convincing him that he was progressing toward total communication that contained more and more of its presurgical characteristics.

Voice and Related Characteristics.   In many areas of clinical work, it is desirable to foster and nurture within our clients a willingness to experiment and literally "play" with their unique abilities to produce speech, voice, and language. The ongoing development and successful refinement of esophageal voice correlates highly with an individual's willingness to take risks, try new suggestions, and experiment, experiment, experiment.

For example, probably every laryngectomee has been disappointed with the reduced loudness of his or her alaryngeal voice. Having a soft voice can cause considerable frustration, particularly in noisy conditions and with listeners who exhibit hearing loss, or with listeners who appear disinterested. Esophageal speakers almost always blame their reduced speech intensity for the problem, when it may or may not be the culprit. Acceptance of those conditions that cannot be changed is obviously one coping strategy. Another strategy might be to address the problem with a willingness to experiment. Experimentation is a desirable clinical tool to use when helping clients realize their potential for changing how loudly or softly they can talk. Why should a laryngectomee not want to talk loudly? After all, a speaking lifetime has been spent in establishing certain patterns. When listeners do not understand or cannot hear, how do laryngeal speakers talk? They talk louder. In the process, laryngeal speakers increase their physical effort. This relationship between effort and intensity is not new to clinicians, but it may be to esophageal speakers and their listeners. It is important that all concerned clearly understand this relationship and ~~view~~ _intensity_ it with a new perspective.

During the refinement of esophageal voice, experimentation with physical effort is essential. Proficient esophageal speakers work on this aspect over a long period of time. If effort were placed on a continuum with excessive effort at one end and too little effort on the other, some interesting associations with esophageal voice would emerge. Too much effort (often closely associated with attempting to talk too loudly) is an area of primary clinical concern. When a speaker fully understands how excessive effort actually reduces intensity/(and often intelligibility), a crucial clinical milepost has been reached. Conversely, too little physical effort may have adverse effects on esophageal insufflation, quality, intensity, and intelligibility. Somehow a balance must be obtained. For many clients, experimentation with various levels of tension and effort while striving to avoid the extremes becomes their long-term clinical goal. Which combination of behaviors yields the greatest intensity, the most pleasing quality, and the most vocal variety is an area of concern. Speaking slowly, quietly, and articulately may afford the patient optimal intelligibility.

A number of other facets of esophageal voice must be considered by the laryngectomee and clinician. For instance (extending vocal range) can be a real challenge for some speakers. Those successful enough to increase range feel a sense of accomplishment and pride. Additional parameters such as (inflection, melody, prosody, and phrasing must be addressed) Individual differences and needs become important considerations. Some clients are seemingly never satisfied, forever listening to and experimenting with the nuances of vocal change. These clients often give the impression of enjoying what they are doing. Others appear to have reached a plateau in their enthusiasm for change. Often, these people seem to have attained a degree of communication proficiency that enables them to be understood consistently across a variety of situations and a number of listeners. These speakers are satisfied with their level of proficiency and fail to recognize and/or care that vocal variety, however viewed, correlates highly with "listenability."

In any discussion of these refinement processes, the clinician's responsibility becomes an issue. How much responsibility should clinicians assume for instilling desire and motivation for change? When and how long do clinicians wait for the desire and motivation to emerge? In this era of patients' rights, it has become very chic for some clinicians to raise the question, "Just who do we as professionals think we are influencing clients' decisions not only as to how they should talk, but how far they should advance on the road to superior esophageal voice?" On the other hand, experienced clinicians can document any number of occasions in which no intervention would have resulted in virtually no change. Thus, a critical balance emerges between laryngectomee and individual clinician. Somehow, much of our clinical competence determines our ability to assess this balance and behave accordingly. Knowing when to react or act becomes crucial. In some instances, chance alone appears to be the most important factor in determining the clinical outcome.

Language Production and Modification.   As mentioned earlier, it seems important for clients to differentiate between speech, voice, and language. It does not take long for alaryngeal speakers to realize which words and phonemic contexts are easier for them to produce. Clinicians can capitalize upon these realizations during individual and group sessions. For example, many clients become aware that the phoneme /h/ is difficult to produce. It would be interesting to know how and where they achieve this understanding. This concept often is an effective entrée into a discussion about context and how essential it is for effective communication. Countless examples abound, but usually someone from the group mentions that an /h/ sound is absent in a cockney dialect and that Professor Henry Higgins of "My Fair Lady" fame omitted /h/ sounds. After such a discussion, the inability by most to produce an /h/ seems less important because the group members have invariably gained a whole new perspective, not nearly as negative as when the discussion began. Refer to chapters 3 and 11 for additional comments on the /h/ sound.

Contextual cues also begin to take on new light and might well lead to appropriate discussion of hearing acuity and hearing loss. In this instance, the nature of the counseling and information provided might be very similar to that which would occur during a discussion with the hearing impaired.

Many clients report that over time they have reduced considerably the number of words in an utterance. It is not uncommon for some esophageal speakers to view this reduction in word output as positive. They may believe that much of what they thought was important or essential to say was superfluous, maybe even irrelevant. Others consider themselves better listeners who do not need to be as verbal as they once were.

Some clients develop fears associated with production of specific sounds or words. Anticipation and expectancy behaviors become learned and evolve in ways similar to those of individuals who stutter. It is amazing how rapidly some of these fears develop. A few clients have demonstrated well-established patterns of word substitution or circumlocution, with interesting consequences. In the extremes, some of these word fears may actually result in a reluctance to speak or a reduction of talking time. When these behaviors occur, it may be necessary for clinicians to involve a variety of listeners to help institute change. A first step for these fearful speakers is to be willing to take risks and to produce the feared sounds or words. Again, the value of group support must be mentioned. In almost every instance, the speaker must become convinced that he or she is capable of making listeners understand what he or she is saying. The speaker rarely will accept one person's word, whether it be from a professional or otherwise. The most potent reinforcement appears to be when the speaker literally becomes convinced. The clinical challenge is to determine what procedures can be utilized to maximize the likelihood that self-reinforcement will occur. Surely, this type of challenge causes clinical work to be exciting.

Generally, the modification of avoidance behavior and the increase of talking time are basic to almost all clinical effort. Changes in these areas take time and must be considered part of long-term goals. Although some clients may take a long time to progress, their slowly acquired behavior will likely be more resistant to change and be established as more permanent.

One index of progress is the degree to which the client is saying what he wants to say when he wants to say it. An honest answer to the question, "Are you talking as much as you want to?" becomes a barometer that reflects change over a variety of speaking situations and over time.

Discussion about this question provides fertile ground for group interaction. Presumably, capable clients are utilizing these group discussions to practice other vocal changes described previously.

Because some clinicians have been taught not to instruct clients to attempt a task unless a rationale is provided, reasons for modifying avoidance behavior will be delineated. These reasons can be grouped into two general areas. First, when a client avoids speaking, he or she is depriving himself or herself knowledge about the outcome of his or her speaking effort. Was the attempt unintelligible? Was the listener really disinterested? Did he or she speak better than anticipated? The responses to these and similar questions generate clinical data that can be used to gain knowledge. In some instances the old axiom "Knowledge of results improves performance" rings true. The second reason for modifying avoidance behavior may be even more relevant or applicable. A relationship exists between avoiding a situation and depriving oneself of an opportunity to practice. In behavioral terms, the client must emit behavior that can be reinforced properly in order to increase the likelihood that the behavior will occur again.

Saying what one wants to say when one wants to say it versus trying not to avoid speaking (or even trying) is another very positive semantic game like was mentioned earlier in this chapter. Approaching change positively seems to have rather strong appeal for some clients, especially those who tend to approach day-to-day living in a positive way.

When clients begin to say what they want to say, other linguistic aspects of their speech change or emerge. Some clients expand their vocabularies, whereas others reduce them with concomitant reductions in the lengths of utterance. Speaking less and in shorter units may not always cause a negative result. Some clients and spouses believe these types of changes actually enhance the quality of interaction.

Implementing some of these vocabulary or utterance-length changes clinically can be quite revealing and challenging. Most clients are surprised at the number of different ways they can express the same thought or bit of information. Having them try to transmit a given message in as few words as possible is one clinical activity. At times, this activity might be viewed as a type of verbal charade. In another exercise speakers could practice expressing a certain idea in a variety of linguistic ways. Some clients report practicing circumlocution in their attempt to find words they believe "will be easier to say." Generally, this roundabout way of speaking results in more constructive outcomes for esophageal speakers than it does for fluency clients who describe histories of word substitution with fairly negative consequences. Thus, another paradox exists in the communicative life of the esophageal speaker: to say it or not to say it.

Hearing acuity and presbycusis are other relevant issues. Campinelli (1964) suggested that hearing function changes in some patients as a result of head and neck surgery. Radiation also may cause changes in hearing. These are valid reasons to argue for a thorough audiological evaluation presurgically, as well as periodic postsurgical evaluations. In some cases, changes in hearing may not become apparent until some time after surgery. Ideally, significant others also should receive audiological evaluations. Proper hearing management can exert profound effects on an individual's communication program. Vanity and reluctance to discuss hearing problems are common among the general population, and laryngectomees appear to be no different from others. For example, one laryngectomee in a clinical program exhibited what appeared to be a fairly limiting degree of hearing loss. His wife reported the usual kinds of frustration (i.e., television too loud, considerable difficulty communicating in the car, her difficulty hearing his esophageal voice, his frustration with not understanding what she said, and his denial of any problem). After a thorough audiological workup, a moderate to severe high-frequency loss was substantiated. When confronted with these data, the client continued to refuse any form of amplification, saying, "I'm not that bad to need a hearing aid." The strongest professional attempt involved encouraging him to try a hearing aid as an adjunct to speech therapy to enable him to monitor his high-frequency stomal blowing. Still he refused. The turning point in this all-too-familiar scenario came after about a year of gentle, and then not so gentle, nudging from fellow laryngectomees. All this time, the client had systematically rejected any suggestions from family and professionals. After witnessing what a hearing aid could do in the case of a newer group member, this client finally succumbed to this positive form of peer pressure. His whole manner changed. He now faced his fellow group members and began interacting in much more mutually satisfying ways. Today he is the group's resident proponent of "getting your ears looked at." This is an example of the group process in action.

Involving Others in the Refinement Process

In many ways, we have already referred to the process of involving others every time a laryngectomee opens his or her mouth. This involvement of others is often stressed with the new user of an artificial larynx. Whenever the instrument is activated, in virtually any new or outside situation, there is a good chance that someone is being exposed to and often educated about this alternative form of communication.

Another area of involving others is to be willing to discuss the "big C"—cancer. Generally speaking, people who learn how to "bring up" or talk about their cancer often seem to have a more rewarding and satisfying pattern of rehabilitation. Most nonlaryngectomees are curious, interested, but often frightened or reluctant to broach the topic of cancer. A laryngectomee's willingness to share information not only provides increased opportunities for practice, but obviously opens the door to education and positive growth for everyone. There is some tried and true philosophy expressed in the sentence, "You can't keep what you don't give away." In other words, the gains made by a laryngectomee become more permanent and meaningful as he or she shares them with others.

Several examples seem appropriate. One cold winter morning one of the clients was waiting for a bus en route to a group speech therapy meeting. Several other people, including a small boy, were waiting on the same corner. Suddenly, the small boy exclaimed in a loud voice, "Mommy, look, there is steam coming out of that man's scarf." While the mother was suffering from embarrassment, the client seized upon the opportunity to educate her and her son about why steam was coming out where it was. When the bus finally arrived, the laryngectomee sat with the boy and his mother, continuing to tell them much more about the real world of a laryngectomee.

Another client was about 6 months postlaryngectomy. His artificial larynx of choice was an intraoral type, the Cooper–Rand. His intelligibility was quite acceptable, but he was extremely reluctant to use the instrument with anyone but his wife and only within the confines of his home. The only other situation in which he would speak with the device was in the one-to-one speech therapy session. He would not attend any group meetings. The pivotal point for him occurred when he was forced to talk with the cashier in his local pharmacy. Upon leaving the drugstore, he was hailed by a woman who had overheard his conversation and who was not only a physician but an otolaryngologist. She had never seen an intraoral artificial larynx, so she was very curious. In this situation, the client felt in a position of authority and he reported spending about half an hour talking with her. From that time on, he showed a marked increase in his talking time and increased progress in developing his esophageal voice. He described that one experience as making a real difference in his life.

Any clinician who has worked with laryngectomees could relate a number of similar anecdotes. Why things happen the way they do and what leads to what are often unanswerable questions. Obviously, many such situations cannot be explained or even contrived. Clinically, it seems worthwhile to encourage clients to take advantage of opportunities and to create opportunities in order to relate their experiences to others.

DISMISSAL

Consideration of when to dismiss a client from a formal management program raises a number of questions and issues. Many practitioners have little experience in this area, probably because so many clients never progress to the point of warranting dismissal. In some programs, there are loosely defined or even nonexistent criteria for terminating therapy. Usually, there are new clients and demands for new services. In other instances, clients cease to participate and simply disappear.

The action of following patients who previously attended therapy also raises some interesting issues and represents a highly desirable aspect of any program. In almost any profession, it seems that more energy could be devoted to the followup of clients.

When it comes to dismissal, it is often difficult to generalize. There are as many needs being met in a program as there are clients. The variety and appropriateness of referral options also may affect the decision to dismiss. Ideally, dismissal issues, are part of an ongoing program planning and should be considered jointly by client and clinician. For some people, termination of formal treatment can represent a positive milepost and be presented as part of the process of change. For other clients, some dependencies may develop that necessitate a gradual phasing away from the formal program. In most cases, some referral to or some involvement in a support program long before the actual dismissal decisions are made can be beneficial. Each situation is unique so that individual planning is strongly encouraged. See chapter 8 for a more comprehensive discussion about dismissal criteria.

Many years ago at a rehabilitation conference, John Snidecor presented some interesting ideas about dismissal issues and support groups. He contended that involvement in support groups should not represent lifetime commitments. He thought it was important for laryngectomees and their significant others to resume social activities that were similar to those they enjoyed presurgically. He believed that too much association with other laryngectomees could lose its effectiveness over time and even create problems. Without doubt, there are many situations in which the postsurgical options have enriched lives far beyond what they were prior to the operation. The theme remains the same: each individual's needs are unique and must be related and planned for accordingly. Such a theme is basic to any refinement process.

REFERENCES

Bryngelson, B. (1966). *Clinical group therapy*. Minneapolis, MN: Denison & Co.
Campinelli, P. A. (1964). Audiological considerations in achieving esophageal voice. *Eye, Ear, Nose, and Throat Monthly, 43*, 76-80.

Duguay, M. J. (1986, February). Using speech aids. In W. H. Perkins & J. L. Northern (Eds.), *Seminars in speech and language: Current strategies of rehabilitation of the laryngectomized patient, 7*(1), 13–29. New York: Thieme Inc.

Mendelson, J. H., & Mello, N. K. (1985). *Alcohol use and abuse in America.* Boston: Little Brown.

Robertson, N. (1988). *Getting better: Inside Alcoholics Anonymous.* New York: William Morrow.

Shanks, J. C. (1986, February). Evoking esophageal voice. In W. H. Perkins & J. L. Northern (Eds.), *Seminars in speech and language: Current strategies of rehabilitation of the laryngectomized patient, 7*(1), 1–12. New York: Thieme Inc.

Williams, D. E. (1957). A point of view about "stuttering." *Journal of Speech and Hearing Disorders, 22,* 390–397.

CHAPTER 5

Group Therapy

Shirley J. Salmon and Kay H. Mount

Salmon and Mount contend that therapy in a group setting affords an avenue of treatment different from that of one-on-one treatment. They describe benefits of group therapy and point out that clinicians, patients, and spouses profit from the support offered by group members. Education, speech, support, and social activities appropriate for use with groups are described by the contributing authors and should be of interest to all speech clinicians working with the laryngectomized population.

Study Questions

1. Salmon and Mount favor use of group therapy despite limited availability of research data to justify its value. Why do you agree or disagree with their position?
2. What are two benefits of group therapy? Provide a specific example for each benefit that might occur in your own clinical setting.
3. What are two group activities that can be used to underscore the need for improved intelligibility?

For many years we have considered group therapy an integral part of a communication/rehabilitation program for laryngectomees and spouses. Admittedly, there is a limited amount of research data that justify the efficacy of group treatment; however, such treatment is recognized worldwide as an effective method for changing attitudes and behaviors, as evidenced by the preponderance of support and educational groups in every community. We believe that numerous benefits are derived from group interactions by patients, spouses, and professionals.

Group therapy can be offered independently or in conjunction with individual therapy. The primary difference between the two treatment types is obvious. In individual treatment functional communication activities are often contrived. In group treatment the environment requires communication interaction with more than one person in a natural setting.

Primary benefits derived from group treatment include education of patients, spouses, clinicians, students, and health professionals about ramifications of the disorder through reactive communication; modification of communicative abilities as a necessary part of interaction; and support of patients, spouses, and clinicians in moments of doubt. We are convinced that patients and spouses are the best teachers. Given the opportunity and an accepting environment, they will impart information that is not available elsewhere. Members of the group learn from each other. They compare their communication skills with others in the group and work to be better than average; some compete to be judged most proficient. When a patient's improvement plateaus in individual treatment, transfer to the group often causes him or her to change through interaction with a role model. Within a short time members of the group begin to consider other participants as members of an extended family; thereby, the concerns and problems of each member become important to everyone. When this occurs, patients and spouses understand that they are not alone. The fact that individual problems are shared by everyone also makes it easier for the clinician to cope with the real tragedies (i.e., recurrence of or terminal cancer) experienced by members of the group.

Most of the contributing authors routinely provide group therapy. They were asked to share some of their favorite activities. Their ideas span the gamut of benefits described above. Several of the authors could not resist making introductory comments about group therapy; these remarks are presented first. Specific activities are grouped under their primary goal(s) and follow the comments. The authors are credited for their activities and are quoted directly.

COMMENTS

Lerman

Group therapy techniques have not been sufficiently described in the laryngectomy literature. The majority of laryngectomees are seen in individual therapy. Nevertheless, group therapy can be beneficial. Learning must be transferred outside the individual clinic sessions, and group therapy, although still within the clinic setting, affords that opportunity.

Duguay

As a reader of this section on group therapy, you may find it helpful to recognize that the success of therapy in groups is directly dependent upon the personality of the group leader and the "personality" or makeup of the group. The activities described in this section obviously will work better for some groups and individuals than for others. A wise person once wrote, "Be who you is, 'cause if you is what you ain't, you ain't what you is." Don't try to be someone else in therapy—be you. Adapt these lessons to fit your own style and personality.

In addition, just because a particular lesson fails with one group, it does not mean it will fail with a different group. Do not discard the lesson as useless, but try it with several different groups before you decide to give it up.

Shanks

The group provides a base against which each member can compare his or her own performance. In the presence of a superior speaker, a neophyte can both raise his or her sights and vow, "If he can do it, so can I!" In addition, the group can judge the performance of a particular member. Criticism may be more accepted from a peer than from a professional clinician. In serving as both critic and model, each member can feel that he or she is contributing to the group. More importantly, each person can listen and learn, even when he or she is not speaking. Truly, group speech therapy is far more than a number of individual therapy sessions occurring at the same time!

EDUCATION ACTIVITIES

Diedrich

Activity 1. This activity illustrates to the laryngectomee how external pressure on the pharyngoesophageal (PE) segment may affect intensity, pitch, and duration of esophageal voice.

Divide the group into pairs. Ask Patient A to say /a/ as long as possible and have Patient B time the duration with a stopwatch; note that the duration will be from 1 to 3 s. Next, ask Patient A to locate the vibrating PE segment with his or her index finger while saying /a/. Finally, ask Patient A to produce /a/ as long as possible with varying degrees of finger pressure and have Patient B again time the duration.

Also ask Patient A to try for increased loudness and variations in pitch (inflection) while producing vowels (a,e,i,o,u). Patient B judges whether variations in pitch are noted and whether the esophageal sound is any louder.

If improvement in duration, intensity, or pitch occurs, then without the use of finger pressure, the patient should try to duplicate the effect by tensing the PE segment area or by changing head/neck posture during phonation. If dramatic improvement has occurred with pressure, but is not duplicated without pressure, then a collar or band that provides this pressure should be considered.

Switch roles for Patients A and B.

A simple chart can be devised and distributed so that the observers can easily enter observations and compare results.

Activity 2. This activity demonstrates the usefulness of consonant air injection in increasing the duration of phonation on one air intake.

Pair off the group members. One patient will produce speech; the observer will count the syllables.

The patient is told to do the following:

1. Take an aircharge (insufflate esophageal air).
2. Produce the sounds in each of the following sets:
   A. Vowels a,e,i,o,u. Say as many of each vowel sound as quickly as possible, starting with /a/ (a,a,a . . .). Repeat for each vowel. The observer counts the number of repetitions.
   B. pa,ta,ka,sa. Say as many of each syllable as quickly as possible, starting with /pa/ (papapapa . . .). Repeat for each syllable. The observer counts the syllables.
   C. la,ra,ma,na. Repeat as in B.

If the patient shows a marked increase in the number of syllables in Set B over Sets A and C, then it can be assumed that he or she is using the consonant to assist in the air charge and increase the length (duration) of the esophageal phonation. Some patients may show syllable number increase in Set C over Set A.

Reverse the roles of the paired groups.

The clinician should prepare a chart that can be passed out so that the counts can be entered easily for comparison.

Those patients who do not increase their phonation time may need special attention from the speech clinician on what they can do to learn consonant press injection. Even inhalers can be taught to inject air from consonants.

Martinkosky

Over the years I have found it beneficial to use the midsagittal model of the head to explain the different methods of air injection for alaryngeal speech. The model is also useful to show patients the differences between their pre- and postoperative anatomy. Usually, a group has consisted of newly laryngectomized patients as well as patients laryngectomized as many as 13 years ago. Patients are always interested in finding out how their voice is now produced, how it was produced before, and why they are having certain sensations. This type of session can help patients learn about the importance of the esophagus and the upper esophageal sphincter relative to esophageal voice, controlling reflux, or actually contributing to reflux secondary to a myotomy. Patients with tracheoesophageal puncture may gain further insights into why they are experiencing reflux when they bend over.

Using the midsagittal model of the head to explain articulation and voice in the laryngectomized individual also has proven very beneficial. In a group situation, questions asked by an individual patient can result in insight for the remaining patients who might be too reticent to ask the question themselves. Additionally, some patients' difficulties with certain types of foods can be explained vividly using the midsagittal model of the head since the esophagus is also depicted.

SPEECH ACTIVITIES

Martinkosky

A group activity that I have found very useful is to have the patients, in round-robin fashion, produce individual intelligibility sentences that are in the form of a question. These questions are taken from an original article by Hudgins, Hawkins, Karlin, and Stevens (1947). To be answered, each question must be understood by the listener. Examples of such questions are "What color is grass?" "What country is north of the United States?" "What number comes between 3 and 5?" and "What letter comes after C?"

This activity enables patients to determine which phonemes they need to produce more clearly. Also, they learn how well they are understood by people other than their family members. In addition, patients are taught to look carefully at the oral structures of speakers and to appreciate the benefits of speech reading from both the listeners' and the speakers' points of view. Language stimulation cards, such as those found in aphasia kits, are used to elicit picture descriptions from patients who are illiterate.

Lerman

Most groups are heterogeneous. The following group activity takes heterogeneity into account, but is designed for the more advanced esophageal and artificial larynx speakers.

The primary goal is intelligibility; however, each person may have an individual goal to achieve (e.g., rate, phrasing, articulation). Members must evaluate their own performances as well as the performances of other participants; this activity includes family or significant others.

All the participants are told to listen to what each person is saying as well as how he or she says it. They are to evaluate intelligibility and whether the speaker is achieving his or her goals.

One person is selected (or volunteers) to start the activity by stating what his or her goals are during the session. When he or she has finished, the group is asked to evaluate only the intelligibility. The individual also is asked to evaluate his or her own intelligibility. Each person is given the opportunity to state his or her goals and participate in the evaluation process.

Following the statements of goals and the judgments of intelligibility, the group members participate in other activities, such as conversing over the telephone, taking turns reading aloud from books, discussing specific news or sporting events, and sharing in question-and-answer periods. During these talk periods each person evaluates whether he or she is meeting individual goals for the session, which include overall intelligibility. Also, each person is evaluated by the group.

The purpose of such a group session is not to compete with others, but to be able to realistically monitor oneself and to help other group members. These are the efforts that should be rewarded by the group members and the clinician.

Carpenter

Many speakers mistakenly assume that greater loudness is required when talking against noise. Unfortunately, their attempts at increasing intensity can be ineffective or, worse, detrimental to their speech. They do not appear to realize that the issue is intelligibility rather than audibility, and that other strategies may be more useful in this context. The purpose of the following activity is to determine which speech strategies may be helpful when trying to talk against noise.

Under the guidance of the clinician, the group first lists three to five strategies that could be tried to make their speech more understandable in noise. One (or more) of the group members is then asked to use these strategies one at a time while reading aloud against a noisy background. The clinician provides several printed sets of comparable speech samples for the task, with 10 sentences (or words embedded in a carrier phrase) in each set. One set is used for each speaking condition.

The first set represents the standard and is to be read in a natural speech pattern with no visual cues provided (i.e., the rest of the group is not allowed to watch the speaker). Each subsequent set is produced using one of the recommended strategies. Instructions for the remaining sets could include the following:

- Use a natural pattern, but add visual cues
- Increase loudness (without visual cues)
- Reduce rate (without visual cues)
- Exaggerate articulation (without visual cues)

The speech stimuli can include phonetically balanced words; rhyming words; and words that differ in terms of high-frequency usage, redundancy, or level of abstraction. Interfering noise can be generated with recorded music or radio talk shows.

As the speaker reads each set of sentences or phrases, other group members try to transcribe the samples. After all samples have been presented, the transcriptions are scored for accuracy ($n/10$, where $n =$ the number of correct responses) and averaged per set. These intelligibility values are then used to compare the standard with the other conditions, with discussion addressing the pros and cons of each strategy.

Where speech skills within the group differ substantially, it may be more appropriate to use a variety of speakers to present the sentences or phrases for each set. This variation can prove more complex, but assures a more representative outcome. Adjustments also can be made to accommodate groups of various sizes by subdividing as needed. Each subgroup can replicate the complete activity or evaluate different strategies in comparison with the standard sample.

Keith

First, in starting group therapy, each group member should introduce himself or herself to fellow group members. Second, each participant should have a goal to share with the group. The goals should be realistic and in small increments and should not be "to learn to speak."

1. To facilitate relaxation and ease of phonation, have group members warm up with repetitions of /pa/ or a series of vowels.
2. Depending upon the group, I may use voiced/voiceless consonants for stimulus material. While one person is reading or speaking the words, the others may write or say them as perceived (e.g., pay–bay, bat–pat, bee–pea, pit–bit, time–dime, do–two, die–tie, tip–dip). Then discuss the results and how productions can be improved. This same approach may be used with patients using artificial larynges or either type of esophageal voice.

Gilmore

One type of intelligibility problem experienced by artificial larynx and esophageal speakers is their difficulty producing homologous sounds. In this context the term *homologous* refers to the three sets (triplets) of voiceless–voiced–nasal sounds produced at the same place in the oral cavity: labial—/p–b–m/, apical lingual—/t–d–n/, lingua-velar—/k–g–ŋ/. By heightening their acoustic cues—that is, by "popping" (increasing intraoral pressure) the voiceless sounds and prolonging the nasals—speakers can increase their intelligibility dramatically.

Group activities can facilitate the initial teaching and the generalization of these sounds because they provide: (a) baseline and progress measures in formal drills and spontaneous interactions, based on group responses (percentage of auditors perceiving target), from listeners and in situations that more nearly reflect target environments than does the individual therapy mode; (b) modeling from skilled members of the group; and (c) reinforcement with spontaneous peer reactions. Moreover, these types of group activities are effective maintenance programs for clients who have completed therapy and might otherwise relax their articulatory precision.

The clinician can develop a useful collection of stimulus/training material on 3 × 5 cards for these activities. The following "sets" are recommended:

A. Each of the following sounds presented on a separate card in orthographic form, large enough to be seen across a group therapy room: p, b, m, t, d, n, k (ck), g, ng.
B. Each triplet group of sounds on a separate card: p–b–m, t–d–n, k–g–ng.
C. Each word on a separate card: toe, dough, doe, no, know, rack, rag, rang, and so forth.
D. Triplet word sets, each set on a separate card: toe–dough–no, rack–rag–rang, backer–bagger–banger, pie–buy–my, and so forth.

E. Two-word contexts (to facilitate auditor identification): bread dough, said no, big toe, eat pie, and so forth.

The difficulty of the activity can be adjusted to the client's (clients') degree of proficiency and need for positive reinforcement/success by increasing the cues available to the listeners. The following order represents recognition tasks of increasing difficulty:

1. A card from Set D (triplet word set) is shown and the listener(s) asked to identify which one of the three words was said.
2. A card from Set B (triplet sound card) is shown and a randomly drawn word having one of those sounds (from Set C) is identified by the listener(s).
3. The target sound is presented in a facilitating two-word context (as in Set E) and the listener identifies the word.
4. A card from Set B (triplet sound card) is shown and a randomly drawn sound from that triplet (Set A) is identified by the listener(s).
5. Any set of cards can be "dealt" randomly to the group members and identified by any listener(s).

Shanks

An opening icebreaker may consist of taking roll, wherein each person responds by saying his or her name or some tone ("uh," "aye," "tie," or "here"). Reciting numbers (counting), letters (alphabet), or words (days, months) can be done first in unison, then in predictable sequence (around a circle/table/group), and finally in an unpredictable sequence. (I may point a fast finger randomly to heighten anxiety in subsequent speakers.) Voluntary phonation is the goal.

The clinician can probe the vocal skill of vowel prolongation by waving his or her arms like a conductor to have all speakers start the sound /a/ at the same time. The clinician can consecutively raise fingers (one, two, etc.) at a 1-s rate for each person to assess his or her own maximum duration of phonation.

Another activity involves having the patients try to say the "impossible" /h/ sound. We teach from the premise that perception of /h/ is enhanced as the speaker tries to make a lingua-velar (not glottal) /h/. In effect, this is akin to a linguapalatal fricative [ç], a German "ich laut" (as in "ich habe"), a linguauvular /χ/ Hebrew consonant ("as in chutzpah")", or a prolonged fricative produced with the /k/ articulatory position. The speaker also may enhance the /h/ perception by increased stomal air expulsion, or by stress features (longer, louder, higher pitched vowel). It is unfair to utter an /h/ word either by itself or in a sentence with contextual clues (e.g., "I comb my hair"). Instead, we use a carrier phrase (e.g., "I can say _____"). Thus the target word "hair" is paired with "air," then with "care." Uttering minimal pairs permits listeners' judgments to exceed chance perception with better speaker articulation.

Finally, the same stress features noted above may come together in group singing. At any given time, half the group members are "singing" while the other half are injecting air into the esophagus to join the singing. Such an activity has been used as warm-up or to begin a club meeting. Some musical selections that have become standard for certain clubs include "Do-Re-Mi" from *Sound of Music,* the "Whiffenpoof Song," "O Tannenbaum," or "Row, Row, Row Your Boat." Some clubs have developed meaningful parodies. The following can be sung to "My Bonnie Lies Over the Ocean":

> My larynx is no longer with me.
> I breathe through a hole in my neck.
> There are other good ways of talking,
> So I say to myself, "What the heck?"
>
> Give me, give me, give me a voice I can use.
> Give me, give me, give me a voice I can use.
>
> I found me a pretty good teacher
> Who told me what I have to do.
> Now I'm an esophageal speaker,
> And I can out-talk even you!
>
> Give me, give me, give me a voice I can use.
> Give me, give me, give me a voice I can use.

Duguay

The most important factor influencing alaryngeal speech intelligibility is articulation. Consequently, I always try to include an articulation drill or exercise in my group sessions. The following contrasting-pairs exercise can be used with groups that have individuals with a wide range of skills. It can be used in groups composed of artificial larynx users, advanced esophageal speakers, and those who can phonate only at a single word level. The reader should realize that good group therapy is actually good individual therapy that is carried on in a group setting.

I begin by writing the following words on the chalkboard (or I distribute them on a handout). One might use only one phoneme pair per activity (e.g., all /f/ vs. /v/ contrasts) or a variety of sound pairs (e.g., fan, van; face, vase; chain, Jane; chin, gin; cap, cab; cup, cub).

I indicate why the pairs are different (i.e., voiced/voiceless), and the group members practice the word pairs individually. A practice clue is to prolong the vowel in the voiced member of the pair. If the group lends itself to doing so, members can play in teams. One team member says one of the words in a contrasting pair, and the other team tries to guess which of the words he or she said. The listening team "votes by majority" for Word 1 or Word 2. A score is kept to decide the winning team. If team play is not appropriate for a group, simply ask for hands to be raised after asking, "How many think he said Word 1 . . . Word 2?" Be sure to provide individual help if the group chooses the incorrect word. Conventional cues that you provide in "normal" articulation therapy can be used to assist correction.

To increase the complexity of the drill, increase the length of the utterance and have each person produce the target at his or her level of competence. Examples include "A new fan/van"; "My red face/vase"; "A pretty chain/Jane"; "Hold onto your chin/grin"; "It looks like a cap/cab"; "A very large cup/cub." The person who can say only one word per air charge needs to say only the one contrasting word, whereas an individual who can say two, three, or all four words per air charge can respond at his or her level of activity.

A variation of this drill is to incorporate articulation with stress and juncture by contrasting the following word pairs: seem or, see more; that's ink, that sink; brief E, brie fee; grate ale, grey tail. Again, the team or group will identify by number which two-word phrase they heard.

If the group seems to enjoy this type of exercise, another variation is to use the following and other similarly constructed stimulus word pairs: that table, that's able, that sable, that able, that's sable.

You might also challenge group members as a homework assignment to bring in their own word lists to stump the other team. Keep it light. Keep it fun. And be sure not to embarrass any participant. Provide whatever help and verbal assistance necessary to protect each member of your group.

Keith

Teaching patients how to stress specific words within phrases or sentences can be accomplished by encouraging changes in loudness or pitch. The clinician provides lists of stimulus material, such as the following, and asks questions to elicit the response with appropriate stress.

Stimulus List	Clinician's Questions
Bob wants coffee.	Who wants coffee?
Bob wants *coffee.*	What does Bob want?
Bob *wants* coffee.	Does Bob want coffee or not?

SUPPORT ACTIVITIES

Strasser

A group with spouses only can be very helpful to those involved. Before starting the discussion or conversation, however, check that no laryngectomee has slipped in!

When such a group meets, I explain first why this meeting has been arranged. This meeting might be the only place for a spouse to share problems and admit changes in his or her spouse. Have each spouse tell his or "story." Remember that spouses of well-rehabilitated laryngectomees often forget the difficulties they encountered right after the operation. The group members do not want to complain, but if you are lucky, they all will be eager to talk. Perhaps you know one spouse of a laryngectomee who is rehabilitated well enough that you can ask the spouse directly in front of the group, "What in the beginning was the biggest problem?" In my experience, as soon as one spouse dares to say, "It is terrible; I do not know how to handle this situation," then many others speak up and agree. I have had some spouses ask me, "How can you still work with laryngectomees? I can only stand my husband when I go on vacation for 2 weeks, three times a year, and I go alone!"

SOCIAL ACTIVITIES

Haroldson

Divide the group into pairs of one laryngectomee and one nonlaryngectomee. Encourage them to interview each other, finding out as much as they can. After 10 to 20 min, reassemble the group and have members take turns sharing whatever information has been learned. Most people enjoy this type of activity, as a variety of objectives can be realized. It also allows for a considerable range of speaking proficiency and variety.

Bosone

The purpose of the activity called "bean spitting" is to teach laryngectomees to use intraoral air for activities normally requiring respiratory air (e.g., speech articulation and spitting). Enough uncooked, rinsed, and dried navy beans are required to provide each participant with a handful. The participants are seated in a circle about 6 ft from a large container, such as a trash basket, which has been placed in the center of the circle. By taking turns, each person tries to spit one bean into the trash basket. After one or two rounds of taking turns, everyone practices at will. The activity is often interrupted to have one particularly skilled "spitter" demonstrate his or her prowess. Bean spitting is a good ice-breaker for new or normally more formal groups. It usually generates hearty laughter, and it emphasizes an exceedingly important function for laryngectomees in training for any form of speech.

REFERENCE

Hudgins, C. V., Hawkins, J. E., Karlin, J. E., & Stevens, S. S. (1947). The development of recorded auditory tests for measuring hearing loss for speech. *Laryngoscope, 57,* 57–89.

CHAPTER 6

Tracheoesophageal Puncture: General Considerations

Stanley J. Martinkosky

Martinkosky offers a clear explanation of the basic differences between conventional esophageal speech and esophageal speech following tracheoesophageal puncture. He reviews the history of surgical–prosthetic procedures and the contributions of Singer and Blom to postlaryngectomy voice restoration. Clinicians will appreciate his detailed step-by-step procedures for counseling those who are candidates for tracheoesophageal puncture. His thorough account of how to fit voice prostheses and tracheostoma valves includes a discussion of their individual advantages and disadvantages.

Study Questions

1. What supplies should the patient take home from the hospital following a tracheoesophageal puncture?
2. How soon after a patient has undergone a tracheoesophageal puncture only should he or she be fitted with the prosthesis?
3. What results would you expect during an air insufflation test from the patient who requires the puncture only?
4. What emergency procedures should a patient follow when his or her voice prosthesis comes out during the night?

For those of us who toiled in the area of alaryngeal speech prior to 1979, Singer and Blom's introduction of the tracheoesophageal puncture voice-restoration procedure was met with great enthusiasm. Despite our best efforts, we were continually frustrated that only 30–40% of our laryn-gectomized patients ultimately developed conversational esophageal speech. Fortunately, use of the artificial larynx was fairly well accepted; however, many patients also wished to develop conversational esoph-ageal speech.

Some of us were aware of Damsté's (1958) methods for working with patients who had developed pharyngeal speech, presumably because of excessively tight pharyngoesophageal (PE) constriction. However, otolaryngologists were not routinely performing myotomies on patients failing to develop esophageal speech. Furthermore, no literature was available relating pre- and postmyotomized patients and their ability to develop esophageal speech. Thus, speech–language pathologists, otolaryngologists, and laryngectomized individuals are grateful to Singer and Blom for their persistence in developing this procedure. Their work has enabled a much larger group of patients to develop fluent conversa-tional esophageal speech.

CONVENTIONAL ESOPHAGEAL SPEECH VERSUS ESOPHAGEAL SPEECH VIA TRACHEOESOPHAGEAL PUNCTURE

As early as 1959, Van den Berg and Moolenaar-Bijl theorized that the neoglottis for esophageal voice functioned in an aerodynamic manner similar to the way in which the vocal folds functioned. Both Damsté (1958) and Rubin (1959) clearly showed a mucosal wave existing at the neoglottis just as it is observed in the vibratory movement of normal vocal folds. This work was recently substantiated by Moon and Weinberg (1987), who concluded that fundamental frequency modulation by tracheoesophageal puncture (TEP) speakers is apparently always medi-ated on an aerodynamic basis.

The TEP voice restoration procedure is based on a sound physio-logical foundation since it provides the speaker with a greater and more powerful air supply for activating and maintaining the vibration of the PE segment than that which is available to the traditional esophageal speaker. In conventional esophageal speech, the air supply is injected into the esophagus. The average capacity of the esophageal reservoir is limited to 80 cc (Van den Berg & Moolenaar-Bijl, 1959). Since the tonicity of the PE segment also determines the degree to which air exits the esophagus during esophageal phonation, this injected air can be depleted very quickly. In contrast, the TEP speaker has available the air supply from the normal pulmonary support system for use during phonation.

Diedrich (1968) provided one of the most comprehensive overviews of the mechanism for esophageal speech. By using his breakdown of this mechanism, we can compare it with the TEP voice restoration mechanism. The first aspect to be considered is air intake. With conventional esophageal speech, the basic task is to inflate the esophagus through injection or inhalation with 80 cc of air, the maximum capacity of the esophagus. Conversely, the TEP patient has 400–1,000 cc of air per breath to drive the neoglottis. The TEP patient's air volume does not depend on the maximum capacity of the esophagus as in standard esophageal speech, but instead depends on tidal volume, resistance of the voice prosthesis, and tonicity of the PE segment (Moon & Weinberg, 1987). In terms of air intake, the method used in standard esophageal speech has to be taught and is not "natural," whereas the normal inhalation for speech used by the TEP patient is a close approximation to that used prior to laryngectomy, as substantiated by the fact that the patient who uses the tracheostoma valve following TEP does so naturally and with very little training.

Although the airflow rates during phonation are analogous for both the standard esophageal and the TEP patients, the important variable is the greater volume of air available to the TEP patient (Moon & Weinberg, 1987). Therefore, TEP speakers have much longer phonation times per breath relative to those of the standard esophageal speaker. As a result, the average TEP patient's speech fluency is better than that of the average esophageal speaker. Although the superior standard esophageal speaker is capable of good fluency, frequently one must practice for months, or even years, to achieve it. The TEP patient often can achieve this within minutes of being fitted with a voice prosthesis.

Because the TEP patient has a much greater volume of air available, overall voice quality, intensity, pitch, and articulation are superior. For more detailed results comparing the voice/speech of TEP patients to that of both standard esophageal speakers and normal speakers, see the articles by Robbins (1984) and Robbins, Fisher, Blom, and Singer (1984).

SURGICAL PROCEDURES

Singer and Blom's (1980) description of the TEP technique was the culmination of nearly 30 years of work by various surgeons to develop a surgical–prosthetic procedure for postlaryngectomy voice restoration.

An excellent historical overview was written by Blom and Singer in 1979. In this history of surgical–prosthetic approaches, they described the initial attempts by Conley, DeAmesti, and Pierce (1958) and Asai (1972) to shunt tracheal air to the esophagus. In 1972 Taub and Spiro introduced the Voicebak voice prosthesis, which shunted the tracheal air through a fistula in the esophagus, and in 1978 Sisson, Bytell, Becker, McConnel, and Singer described a similar device.

Another surgical reconstructive technique was introduced in 1969 by Staffieri (cited in Blom & Singer, 1979). Staffieri attempted to surgically construct a mucosal neoglottis that would vibrate when activated by tracheal airflow into the esophagus, but that also would prevent aspiration during swallowing. This and similar procedures were successful for some patients. Widespread application of these techniques never occurred, however, due to stenosis of the shunts, chronic swallowing problems, and difficulties related to operating on irradiated tissue.

In 1977, Amatsu, Matsui, Maki, and Kanagawa developed a surgical technique in which a tracheal flap of tissue was tubed to form a mucosal tunnel connecting the esophagus and trachea. Although good results were reported with this technique, tract stenosis and aspiration of liquids during swallowing were experienced by some patients.

TRACHEOESOPHAGEAL PUNCTURE TECHNIQUE

Singer and Blom (1978) attempted the Amatsu procedure on a number of patients. As a result of their experiences, they developed the TEP voice restoration technique. This procedure was designed to alleviate fistula tract stenosis and aspiration difficulties. Both of these chronic problems were overcome by introducing a unique one-way air valve called the *duckbill*. This duckbill voice prosthesis simultaneously keeps the fistula tract open, prevents aspiration during swallowing, and allows passage of tracheal airflow into the esophagus. The valve opens under positive pressure during expiration and closes by elastic recoil. For a complete description of the Singer–Blom technique, see the original 1980 article.

The major difference in today's procedure from that described in the original article is that the catheter is no longer threaded up through the fistula and through the nose. Currently, following puncture, the catheter (usually a 14 French [Fr.]) is directed downward into the esophagus. Use of the catheter in this manner has the advantage of angling the fistula slightly downward and eliminating potential irritation to the nasal mucosa. Also, the catheter can serve as a feeding tube when the patient has undergone the TEP as part of the primary laryngectomy

(Hamaker, Singer, & Blom, 1985) or a myotomy at the time of the TEP procedure.

Selection Criteria

In 1980, Singer and Blom reported their initial 2-year experience employing TEP for reestablishment of voice after total laryngectomy with 60 postlaryngectomized patients. They stressed the importance of careful patient selection, with particular emphasis on patient motivation, ability to care for the stoma and prosthesis, adequate stoma size and position, and insufflation testing to assess pharyngeal constrictor muscle tonicity. Also, they recommended that patients with a history of fistula, stricture, or flap reconstruction, be assessed by barium esophagram. Since that time a number of articles have addressed the long-term results of the Singer–Blom speech rehabilitation procedure (Blom, Singer, & Hamaker, 1981; Schuller, Jarrow, Kelly, & Miglets, 1983; Wetmore, Johns, & Baker, 1981; Wetmore, Krueger, Wesson, & Blessing, 1985).

Andrews, Mickel, Hanson, Monahan, and Ward (1987) described the patient characteristics necessary for the TEP procedure as (a) motivation and mental stability, (b) adequate understanding of the anatomy and the mechanics of the prosthesis, (c) adequate manual dexterity and visual acuity to care for the stoma and the prosthesis, (d) no significant hypopharyngeal stenosis, (e) speech production with esophageal insufflation via a properly positioned esophageal catheter, (f) adequate pulmonary reserve, and (g) stoma of adequate depth and diameter to accept the prosthesis without airway compromise.

Complications

In the same article, Andrews et al. (1987) summarized the most common complications of the TEP procedure, including allergic reaction to tape or prosthesis, esophageal preparation, enlarging fistula, stoma stenosis, fistula migration, major cellulitis/infection, stenosis of the esophagus secondary to prosthesis, aspiration of prosthesis, aspiration pneumonia, and death secondary to aspiration.

Complete Assessment of Patient's Candidacy

At a time deemed appropriate by the surgeon and speech–language pathologist, the patient undergoes esophageal insufflation testing (Blom, Singer, & Hamaker, 1985). This testing is done to determine candidacy for TEP and whether a myotomy will be required. In addition to performing well during the esophageal insufflation, the "ideal" patient must exhibit (a) adequate stoma size and configuration for placement of a voice prosthesis without interfering with respiration; (b) a personal desire to undergo the procedure, rather than simply satisfying a spouse's desire; (c) willingness to undergo training for self-care and placement of the voice prosthesis; and (d) adequate manual dexterity and eyesight to enable prosthesis management.

Insufflation Procedure

Prior to insufflating the esophagus, the examiner informs the patient about the procedure and explains that the patient will have a sensation of fullness in his or her throat. At our center, the otolaryngologist usually topically anesthetizes the patient's clearest nostril for insertion of the 14 Fr. Robinson type urethral catheter. He inserts the catheter through the patient's nares and down into the pharyngeal area until it reaches the pharyngoesophageal zone. Then the patient is encouraged to swallow so that the catheter can be moved into the upper esophagus. When the tip of the catheter moves down into the upper esophagus, one can hear the esophageal pressure changes via the catheter as the patient swallows. To ensure that the catheter has gone downward past the base of the tongue, one should routinely look in the patient's mouth to be certain the catheter has not curled in the oropharyngeal area. If the catheter has curled within this area, the patient will exhibit noticeable discomfort, or gag secondary to irritation from the tube.

While holding the catheter securely in place, the examiner connects a Bird Pressure Manometer to the proximal tip. The catheter must be stabilized at this location in the upper esophagus and not be allowed to slide either up or down. The patient is instructed to let his or her mouth relax and open slightly for the production of the vowel /a/ and is cautioned against exhaling vigorously during insufflation. To preclude the accidental backflow of the patient's esophageal contents, the examiner, when performing the insufflation test, should always ensure that the manometer and his or her own head are well above the level of the patient's nose. The examiner then begins to blow air gently into the catheter while monitoring the manometer. As the needle begins to rise between 10 and 40 cm/$H_2$0, activation of esophageal vibration should occur. If esophageal tone is achieved, the pressure reading required to activate/sustain sound is noted, and the patient is asked to produce vowel sounds. If no spasmodic activity is detected, the patient is then asked to utter several functional phrases consisting initially of continuant sounds, such as, "Where are you?" and "How are you?" Following this, the patient is required to produce functional phrases with voiced and voiceless consonants, such as, "What time is it?" "How are you today?"

and "I like chocolate chip cookies." Finally, he or she is asked to count from 1 to 15 while the examiner provides the air supply via the catheter.

During each insufflation, the examiner monitors the pressure at which the patient is able to initiate and/or sustain phonation. If the phonation is sustained during vowels and continuants but not during voiced and voiceless sound production, the examiner tries to encourage phonation with as low a pressure as possible. Low-pressure activation is done to determine whether cessation of phonation is due to (a) insufflation of the esophagus too quickly by the examiner, or (b) difficulty with voiced/voiceless contrasts, or (c) subtle reflexive contraction of the pharyngeal constrictor muscles.

If the patient is able to produce vowels, continuants, voiced/voiceless contrast, and numbers without any hint of reflexive spasm or tightness, it is assumed that he or she will not require a myotomy. More important, if the patient is unable to complete these tasks, even when the manometer rises above 40 to 50 cm/H_2O, it is assumed that a myotomy or a pharyngeal plexus neurectomy (Singer, Blom, & Hamaker, 1986) is indicated at the time of the TEP.

Incidentally, we have had several patients in whom we were unable to place the urethral catheter into the esophagus. When these patients underwent a preoperative modified barium swallow, esophageal stricture was revealed. One should never assume that the patient with a stricture requires a myotomy. In fact, some of our best patients' voices have come from those patients exhibiting some degree of stenosis or stricture. On several patients referred for postoperative strictures, surgeons have performed myotomies. The results were very flaccid esophageal sphincters and unacceptable, breathy voice quality. Thus, it is good to keep in mind that the tonicity of the esophagus caused by the stricture might well enhance the vibratory characteristics of the esophagus.

Other Considerations

In addition to results of the esophageal insufflation test and the decision regarding a myotomy, the patient's stoma size and configuration must be considered prior to TEP. The stoma with a pyramidal shape—that is, a narrow superior aspect and wider inferior aspect—has always been considered the ideal configuration. Other shapes considered acceptable are the elongated or elliptical stoma and the large stoma. Some stomas, no matter what configuration, will need revision if the voice prosthesis is expected to occupy more than 30% of the total area.

Team Approach

The best way to manage a TEP patient is to use a team approach consisting of the surgeon and speech–language pathologist. The patients of otolaryngologists using nurses instead of speech–language pathologists have less chance to succeed. Speech–language pathologists who work alone—removed from the otolaryngology clinic, the otolaryngologists, and other facilities associated with the otolaryngology clinic—also are less able to provide optimal postoperative care.

The patient is under the direct care of his or her surgeon. The surgeon is responsible for deciding when the patient is medically appropriate for evaluation of TEP. For example, the surgeon alone is aware of the extent of the patient's original tumor, the aggressiveness of the tumor, the response of the patient to postoperative radiation therapy, and the patient's general prognosis.

To provide continuity of care, the speech–language pathologist also should be an active member of the team from the preoperative phase of the patient's care through the postoperative follow-up for alaryngeal speech therapy. This role includes being closely involved in the evaluation of the patient's appropriateness for the TEP voice restoration procedure.

When a speech pathologist and surgeon work together, each assumes a supportive role for the other. As described previously, the surgeon typically anesthetizes the patient's nose for the placement of the insufflation catheter and inserts the catheter through the nose, threading it down through the pharynx into the esophagus. The surgeon also is present while the speech–language pathologist performs the esophageal insufflation test, preferably using the oral manometer. Use of the manometer enables the speech pathologist to obtain quantifiable readings of the intraluminal pressure during the insufflation test. Both surgeon and speech pathologist can share their opinions regarding the test results and decide whether the patient's stoma requires revision or enlargement to accommodate the voice prosthesis. Since a given patient might undergo three procedures—the TEP, a myotomy, and a stoma revision—the surgeon must be prepared to explain the need for each to the patient. The speech pathologist also consults with the patient to underscore information provided by the surgeon, and to be sure that the patient understands all aspects of the proposed surgical procedures.

PREOPERATIVE COUNSELING FOR LARYNGECTOMY

Candidates for a TEP procedure are referred by an outside otolaryngologist, hospital, or otolaryngology staff member, or they are self-referred. They may be patients who are being prepared for primary laryngectomy, who are several months postlaryngectomy and postradiation, or who are as much as 5–10 years postlaryngectomy. The sequence of events usually proceeds as follows:

1. The patient is diagnosed as having carcinoma of the larynx, which will necessitate a total laryngectomy with or without neck dissection.

2. The speech pathologist is informed about the patient by the physician.

3. The clinician meets with the patient and the family to explain the dynamics of speech and voice production with and without a larynx. Usually, a midsagittal model of the head and neck is used to demonstrate pertinent anatomy. This model enables the patient and the family to relate more realistically to the implications of the impending surgery.

4. The questions of the patient and the family are answered from a speech–language pathologist's viewpoint. Questions of a medical and surgical nature are referred back to the surgeon. The clinician also informs the patient that he or she will have a nasogastric tube in place for sustenance while the esophagus heals.

5. The clinician explains the method for esophageal insufflation and production of conventional esophageal speech. Again, the midsagittal model of the head and neck is used.

6. Also, the clinician demonstrates the various artificial larynges. At the patient's request, he or she should be allowed to try the larynges. These devices are usually described as backup systems, although mention should be made that many patients use them as their sole means of communication. The clinician advises the patient that since he or she will be swollen immediately following the operation, an intraoral device such as the Cooper-Rand is initially the instrument of choice. Plans are made to evaluate the patient's candidacy for neck-type devices when swelling subsides.

7. The TEP procedure is usually explained last. The midsagittal model of the head is used to position the voice prosthesis so the patient can see its approximate location and mechanical nature as a one-way air valve. Both the duckbill and low-pressure voice prostheses are shown to the patient. The dynamics are explained, and the patient is encouraged to examine the prostheses. Time permitting, the patient and the family may view portions of videotapes that show a variety of patients utilizing artificial larynges, conventional esophageal speech, and tracheoesophageal puncture speech with and without the tracheostoma valve. We believe that videotapes of our own patients are more effective and relevant to our patient population than are those produced commercially.

8. When possible the patient and family are introduced to other laryngectomized individuals of the same gender utilizing representative

    esophageal speech, artificial laryngeal speech, and tracheosophageal speech.

9. When appropriate, the patient is given the brochure about laryngectomy by Keith, Shane, Coates, and Devine (1984), which provides additional information for the patient and the family in preparation for the surgery.
10. Also, we assure our patients that in all of our years at this facility, no patient has ever died undergoing total laryngectomy.
11. An attempt is made to obtain a baseline audiogram, usually consisting of puretone, air and bone, and speech reception thresholds prior to surgery. Sometimes this must be scheduled postoperatively because the patient has already been overloaded with preoperative tests and counseling sessions prior to surgery.
12. The patient's speech and voice are tape-recorded during conversation, vowel prolongations, and production of a list of intelligibility sentences.
13. Information about length and course of hospital stay also is provided (i.e., laryngectomy usually requires approximately a 2-week hospitalization, including the day of surgery and a day in the intensive care unit). The fact that the patient is usually brought to the regular patient floor 2 or 3 days after surgery is emphasized. The patient is informed that he or she probably will have a considerable amount of swelling in the chin and neck area, and initially this will hamper speech articulation. For this reason, the patient will be encouraged initially to utilize a writing pad or magic slate and, later, an intraoral artificial larynx.
14. Finally, the patient is informed that a clinician will come to his or her room within a few days following surgery to assess his or her condition relative to beginning use of the artificial larynx.

POSTOPERATIVE COUNSELING FOR LARYNGECTOMY

The Cooper-Rand artificial larynx is usually brought to the patient's bedside for initial training and familiarization within a day or two following the laryngectomy. Training begins with tube placement and tone control to facilitate functional communication as soon as possible. This is particularly important with patients who are illiterate or are very poor writers. For literate patients the magic slate or writing pad and pencil are provided simultaneously with learning to use an artificial larynx.

    We find it helpful to bring successful alaryngeal speakers to visit the patient postoperatively. Within a week the patient has usually been visited by one using an artificial larynx, one using a voice prosthesis, and one using conversational esophageal speech. They are asked to visit the patient, demonstrate their speaking skills, and answer questions. The voice prosthesis of the TEP speaker is called to the attention of the new laryngectomee. If the visiting speaker is using the tracheostoma valve, it is initially removed and the speaker is asked to occlude the stoma to demonstrate the digital–stomal-occlusion technique. The valve is then reinserted so that automatic stomal occlusion can be observed. When appropriate, each visitor and the newly laryngectomized patient are left alone so they can communicate about their mutual concerns.

The majority of our patients undergo 30 postoperative radiation therapy treatments. During this 6-week period, work with the artificial larynx is scheduled. Therapy sessions are usually provided several times a week in conjunction with radiation therapy visits. A "loaner" artificial larynx is used while assessing the patient's abilities with various types of devices. I am a strong proponent of the dual approach to alaryngeal speech; that is, I believe that every laryngectomized patient should have some type of artificial larynx available either as a primary or backup system. Once the device best suited to the patient has been determined, it is obtained through our hospital patient equipment department. Thus, the cost of the patient's device can be billed directly to hospitalization, and the patient is relieved from ordering the device and completing third-party payment forms. This method also eliminates the possibility that the patient might not order the device due to lack of insurance coverage.

During this postoperative follow-up period, new patients are invited to attend clinic treatment sessions conducted with successful TEP patients. New patients observe voice prosthesis insertion procedures, stoma occlusion practice, and application and use of the tracheostoma valve.

Esophageal speech training is not provided to any patient who expresses an interest in TEP voice restoration. In our experience, patients who have learned to use the air injection technique for conventional esophageal phonation have had difficulty extinguishing this maneuver when they begin to use their new TEP speech.

PREOPERATIVE TEP ORIENTATION

Although all patients have been provided information about the TEP prior to their laryngectomy and have met several TEP patients, each prospective TEP patient is given a detailed explanation of the procedure. Again the midsagittal model of the head and neck proves very beneficial since the placement of the fistula as well as the voice prosthesis can be demonstrated and the entire mechanism explained. This model also facilitates questions and answers regarding anatomic changes following the TEP.

The patient and family also are shown several types of voice prostheses and inserters to become familiar with the manner in which they function. If the patient is to undergo a myotomy and/or a stoma revision, the rationale for these procedures is explained and the pertinent anatomy is discussed. If a myotomy or stoma revision is planned, the patient is advised of appropriate recovery periods that will be needed before he or she can begin tracheoesophageal speech. If the patient is literate, instructions for cleaning and inserting the voice prosthesis may be provided so that the patient begins orientation to care and maintenance of the appliance. In this way, the clinician has the opportunity to assess patient motivation for self-care and maintenance, as well as any reluctance to use the device. The patient's dexterity also can be determined. This training is particularly useful with a patient who requires a family member or health professional to aid in prosthesis removal, insertion, and cleaning.

POSTOPERATIVE TEP ORIENTATION

The patient is seen for the first time postoperatively by the speech pathologist in an examining room at the otolaryngology clinic. Here, suction is available for the speech pathologist if the patient begins to cough or have leakage through the fistula. The presence of the suction device permits the clinician to feel more secure because he or she is prepared for potential respiratory problems.

Required Supplies

Supplies that should be present in the examining room are (a) oral manometer (we use a Bird Model), (b) coudé-tipped 14 Fr. catheter, (c) coudé-tipped 16 Fr. catheter, (d) clear 10 Fr. catheter with the very tip clipped off (to fit within the voice prosthesis itself), (e) voice prosthesis sizing device, (f) viscous lidocaine, (g) hypoallergenic tape, (h) tweezers, (i) suture scissors, and (j) several duckbill voice-prostheses to be used as initial trial voice prostheses (see the appendix at the end of the chapter for a list of supply sources).

Timing

Keep in mind that the patient undergoing TEP only will be coming to the clinic approximately 48 hr after the fistulization. The patient with the TEP plus myotomy will probably go home after 2 days with the 14 Fr. urethral catheter in the fistula and return 2 to 10 days following discharge, depending upon whether the myotomy caused some esophageal tearing. These tears must heal prior to use of a prosthesis for esophageal insufflation. The TEP patient who also had a stoma revision will generally be seen 48 hr after puncture for sizing and fitting of the voice prosthesis; however, stoma occlusion is deferred. Because the stoma area is tender, placement of the thumb to occlude it for phonation is precluded. Finally, the patient who has undergone TEP plus myotomy and stoma revision is discharged 2 days following the puncture, unless a fistula occurs or infection develops. This patient will return to the clinic 2 or 3 days following discharge for voice prosthesis fitting; again, occlusion of the stoma for voicing might be deferred.

Initial Insertion of Prosthesis

Whenever the patient is first seen in the otolaryngology clinic for voice prosthesis placement, the suction catheter is first connected and tested. Next, the speech pathologist or the otolaryngologist removes the sutures that have been holding the catheter in place. These two sutures are usually 3–5 cm lateral to the stoma.

Prior to removing the 14 Fr. catheter from the fistula, the clinician cleans the stoma and tracheal areas with hydrogen peroxide applied around the stoma with cotton swabs. This may require the care of the nurse or otolaryngologist if crusting extends deep into the trachea or if the mucous crusts are so hard that bleeding might occur unless a softening solution such as saline is applied prior to removal.

Testing the Phonatory Mechanism.   The fitting process is begun by explaining the procedure to the patient. The clinician tells the patient that the catheter will be removed and another 16 Fr. soft red coudé-tipped catheter will be placed within the fistula to keep it open or to use with the manometer. (Since some surgeons inflate the urethral catheter balloon slightly rather than stitch it into place, residual air or water from the catheter balloon must be withdrawn using a standard 10-cc syringe before the catheter can be removed.) The replacement catheter is used to assess the patient's capacity to produce voice while the clinician gently insufflates the esophagus and notes the manometric pressure. The manometer allows the clinician to monitor the amount of intraluminal pressure present when esophageal phonation is activated, ceased, or sustained consistently. This is an optimal measure because there is no resistance from a voice prosthesis. The only time there is less resistance in the patient's fistula is when it is completely open (i.e., the patient is inhaling, occluding the stoma with the thumb, and phonating by passing air through the fistula without any catheter or voice prosthesis). This lack of resistance is what the Blom–Singer low-pressure and Bivona low-resistance voice prostheses were designed to approximate.

Using the catheter technique, the clinician can determine whether the phonatory mechanism is functioning properly. He or she also can determine the patient's sensitivity to air passing through the esophagus relative to triggering the regurgitation reflex. The same series of tasks described for preoperative insufflation testing are carried out. Thus, stoma revision patients can be assessed without digital pressure against the stoma.

Sizing. When the clinician has determined that the PE segment is functioning properly relative to airflow and phonation, the patient is informed that the catheter will be removed and a sizing device will be placed within the fistula. The sizing device is essentially a dummy prosthesis with striations enabling the examiner to estimate the length of the voice prosthesis that should be inserted. We have utilized both the Bivona and the Blom–Singer sizing devices. In our opinion, the Bivona device has proved more useful.

Following complete insertion of the sizing device, the clinician gently retracts it, allowing the flange to engage against the anterior wall of the esophagus. He or she notes the number of striations visible on the sizing device and checks the size that corresponds with that number of striations. If the length of the fistula is between striations, or the striation is difficult to visualize, the next longer size prosthesis is recommended, especially at this early stage of sizing. Choosing the shorter prosthesis at this point can result in two potential problems. The voice prosthesis could fit and snap into place but have a great deal of tension on it. This tension could result in slight tissue swelling or dislodgement with patient movement. Also, if the prosthesis does not optimally enter the esophagus even though it appears to do so, then the inner wall of the fistula can dimple down, resulting in spontaneous closure and preventing passage of air through the fistula. Repuncture might then be required.

Inserting. When the correct prosthesis size has been determined, the clinician tells the patient that the sizing device will be removed and the voice prosthesis will be inserted. The angle of the fistula is manifested in the angle of the sizing device; therefore, the clinician must take particular care to follow the same angle when inserting the voice prosthesis as he or she did when inserting the sizing device.

Also, prior to inserting the initial voice prosthesis, the clinician can slide a 16 Fr. coudé-tipped catheter through the fistula to stretch it slightly, making more space for the voice prosthesis within the tender fistula tract. We have used viscous lidocaine on the catheter as a temporary lubricant and topical anesthetic to the area. It takes several minutes for the viscous lidocaine to have the optimal effect. We have also put a small amount of viscous lidocaine on the side of the flange that will rub against the fistula wall as it is inserted. When inserting the voice prosthesis, it essentially is going through two walls, the posterior tracheal wall and the anterior esophageal wall. Usually a definite vibratory sensation is felt via the insertion device when the flange opens into the esophagus. It is important to demonstrate this to the patient because he or she may use excessive force to insert the prosthesis and therefore be unaware of this sensation. This tactile feedback informs the patient that the voice prosthesis is placed correctly. In the initial stage of training, the patient's cough frequently masks any potential auditory feedback from the inserter.

Once the voice prosthesis is placed, the insertion device can be left in the voice prosthesis temporarily to show the patient the angle of his or her tract. This is visualized in a mirror. We prefer the slightly downward angle for the fistula because this downward angle directs the valved prosthesis tip away from the passage of food and liquids. The fistula angle can be redirected slightly downward by tightening the tape on the outer flap of the voice prosthesis in an upward direction.

To remove the inserter we recommend that the patient twirl the inserter while withdrawing it from the voice prosthesis. Otherwise, the friction from the inserter against the inner walls of the prosthesis can result in partial dislodgement. If this happens, the patient may have a false impression that the voice prosthesis is well seated, when in fact the inner aspect of the fistula could stenose due to malpositioning. We recommend that the patient check the seating of the voice prosthesis by tugging gently outward on its strap after completing the insertion process.

Once the voice prosthesis is in place, we ensure that the vent window on the underside of the prosthesis is facing downward toward the tracheal airflow with the strap perpendicular to the stoma and taped in position. We have found the brown Johnson & Johnson Dermiclear Transparent Tape to be quite durable. Other patients prefer either the ½-in. or 1-in. paper tape since it has very light adhesive.

Voicing. With the voice prosthesis in place, we have the patient inhale and, while we occlude the stoma gently, attempt to phonate. Frequently, the patient will overinflate the esophagus and sometimes will not utilize adequate abdominal pressure to activate the airflow optimally. This results in either no voicing due to lack of airflow or overinflation causing excessive pressure between the voice prosthesis and the thumb. We reinstruct the patient and have him or her inhale more appropriately. The clinician occludes the stoma again. If acceptable voicing is produced, the patient is asked to occlude the stoma for voicing. At first, the patient may inhale too deeply, overinflate the esophagus, or push too firmly on the stomal area with the thumb. Pushing too firmly against the prosthesis can cause the airflow port to enter the fistula, or the tip of the prosthesis to touch the posterior wall of the esophagus and impede opening of the duckbill or flapper valve.

If the patient and/or clinician uses optimal stoma occlusion and still produces inconsistent voice, the clinician should connect the manometer to a 10 Fr. pediatric catheter. By cutting off the very tip of this catheter, the catheter can be inserted into the voice prosthesis. The clinician can blow air through the voice prosthesis and into the esophagus and eliminate digital contact against the stoma. If esophageal phonation is obtained while using the catheter through the voice prosthesis, but not obtained with stoma occlusion, this usually indicates that only a small space exists between the tip of the voice prosthesis and the posterior wall of the esophagus. The result is contact of the voice prosthesis tip against the esophageal wall, preventing opening of the duckbill valve. When this occurs try (a) utilizing an even lighter contact on the stoma, (b) simultaneously occluding the stoma and angling the voice prosthesis downward, or (c) changing to a low-pressure/resistance voice prosthesis which has no extended tip on it. The patient also would be a candidate for the tracheostoma speaking valve, which eliminates the need for digital pressure to occlude the stoma.

Once problems of fitting the prosthesis have been solved, speech tasks can be introduced. Our patients progress from the vowels, to continuant-type phrases, and then to functional phrases frequently spoken around the home. The patients are encouraged to use the optimal pattern of short inhalation, occlusion of stoma, and then speech.

A practice exercise that we utilize consists of intelligibility sentence lists by Hudgins, Hawkins, Karlin, and Stevens (1947). The advantage of these sentences is that they are simple questions and require only one-word answers. Furthermore, they do not require that every individual phoneme be articulated precisely for the speaker to be functionally intelligible. At this stage we are primarily interested in functional communication and overall speech intelligibility, not complete phonemic accuracy. Practice with these questions requires intelligible speech if the listener is to respond with the correct answers. Immediate feedback concerning the speaker's intelligibility is provided by the listener's ability to answer.

Precautions. After the initial session and fitting of the voice prosthesis, the patient is given a "safety" catheter, usually a 14 Fr. coudé-tipped one. This catheter is to be used in the event that the voice prosthesis comes out prior to the next session. In such an instance, the patient is to insert the catheter into the fistula and return to the hospital without danger of aspiration or of having the fistula close. Of course, the patient practices inserting the catheter prior to going home. This also prepares the groundwork for steps required during routine placement of the voice prosthesis, since we will have the patient place the catheter each time the voice prosthesis is removed. The larger 16 Fr. catheter is used in combination with the regular voice prosthesis. An 18 Fr. catheter is routinely inserted in the fistula to dilate it prior to insertion of the Blom–Singer low-pressure or the new Bivona ultra–low-resistance voice prostheses. A 20 Fr. catheter must be used prior to inserting the 20 Fr. Bivona voice prostheses.

Usually, the patient is scheduled to return to the clinic within a day or two if he or she lives nearby, or possibly after the weekend or the next week if the distance is farther. Some patients remain in the hospital and can be followed daily. Other patients stay in the hospital motel unit so they can return every day or two for follow-up training.

Follow-Up Training for Self-Insertion of Prosthesis

During the second session with the patient, we review the steps we will practice and then have the patient remove the voice prosthesis. We show the patient how to grip the prosthesis strap and pull firmly outward until it dislodges. We caution that he or she will hear a strange popping as it dislodges. The patient has the catheter ready so that as soon as the voice prosthesis is removed, he or she can immediately place the tip of the catheter in the fistula and insert it a distance of 5–10 cm. At times, removal of the voice prosthesis causes coughing, mucus expectoration, and minor saliva leakage from the fistula, which can obscure the location of the fistula site. To remedy this problem caution the patient to inhale gently to increase the negative pressure in the esophagus so that mucus in the fistula is sucked inward to the esophagus. With the patient positioned in front of a mirror and a light focused directly on the stoma, the patient gently inserts the 16 Fr. catheter. Some patients are very cautious when inserting the catheter. The clinician must help these patients overcome fear by gently guiding and reinforcing their efforts to insert the catheter.

With the catheter in the fistula, the patient prepares the replacement voice prosthesis for insertion. The patient removes the catheter and then places the tip of the voice prosthesis in the fistula at the proper angle. The voice prosthesis is inserted into the fistula until the sensation or sound of the retention flange opening in the esophagus is detected.

Desensitization. Some patients learn prosthesis insertion readily, but others may take weeks to become desensitized to this procedure and gain confidence and independence in voice prosthesis insertion. Most patients will be able to remove the catheter and place the tip of the voice prosthesis in the fistula; however, when the flange meets the fistula opening, some patients "freeze" and appear unable to push the voice prosthesis any further. When this occurs reassure the patient and remind him or her to relax as you gently assist pushing inward on the insertion device. Also, remind the patient to monitor the sensation of the flange opening into the esophagus as the prosthesis is pushed into the fistula.

Precautions. We do not like to practice placing, removing, and replacing the voice prosthesis too often during the initial sessions due to tissue irritation and swelling at the fistula site. Overpractice can result in discomfort for the patient, possible bleeding at the site, and a negative attitude. We would rather have the patient tolerate a nonfunctioning prosthesis occluded by mucus for a day or so than have him or her remove the prosthesis too frequently. This is another reason for the patient to have a backup system, such as an artificial larynx, which provides the patient with an alternative mode of communication while he or she is learning and adapting to use of the voice prosthesis.

Practice. At each successive session the above steps are repeated. As he or she becomes more confident in the insertion process, the patient also begins experimenting with different patterns of stoma occlusion, including the use of different fingers and hands.

Selection of Optimal Prosthesis Type. A change from the duckbill to the low-pressure or low-resistance voice prosthesis occurs earlier for some patients than for others. We ordinarily do not change to a low-pressure or low-resistance prosthesis until we believe the patient has confidence and consistency in the ability to care for and maintain a duckbill-type voice prosthesis. Since the esophageal tips of the low-pressure or low-resistance voice prostheses are shorter and open-ended, they scrape through the fistula site rather than sliding through like the duckbill prosthesis. Therefore, we prefer to allow the fistula to mature and the patient to have the experience of inserting a duckbill-type prosthesis numerous times prior to converting to a low-pressure or low-resistance voice prosthesis.

Prior to use, each voice prosthesis should be checked to ensure that the tip is functional. Duckbill-type voice prostheses should be squeezed gently behind the flange so that the tip opens. If at first it does not, one can gently prod the tip to facilitate release. In the case of the low-pressure or low-resistance voice prostheses, the valve should be squeezed to check that the flap opens and closes. In some of these prostheses we have found the flap inverted. It is pushed or sucked into the opening in the voice prosthesis and must be repositioned with the inserter. If the flap is not correctly seated, liquids will run back through the prosthesis when the patient swallows. With the duckbill-type voice prosthesis, the pressure inside the esophagus sometimes can hold the duckbill closed. This is not the case with the low-pressure voice prosthesis. Liquid will take the path of least resistance under the positive intraluminal pressure created during swallowing.

The fistula sites in some patients tend to appear as small slits rather than nice round fistulas. A patient with a slit-type fistula benefits from using a prosthesis with a duckbill tip rather than a low-pressure or low-resistance tip. When attempting to insert a low-pressure or low-resistance voice prosthesis, the patient can easily let it slip from the opening of the fistula downward against the tracheal wall. This stimulates coughing and increases the chance that the voice prosthesis is accidentally aspirated. Should a patient with this slit-type fistula require a low-pressure or low-resistance voice prosthesis, the patient will need to place an 18 or even 20 Fr. catheter into the fistula prior to insertion of the prosthesis. If these larger catheters are left in the fistula for 5–10 min, even the slit-type fistula usually will remain open long enough for the patient to remove the catheter and quickly insert the prosthesis.

Low-pressure or low-resistance voice prostheses are made by both of the major voice prosthesis manufacturers. Choice of a low-pressure or low-resistance prosthesis or of a duckbill prosthesis depends upon the preference and experience of the examiner and the needs of the patient.

Insertion of Low-Pressure or Low-Resistance Voice Prosthesis. For patients who use a low-pressure or low-resistance voice prosthesis, we dilate the fistula with the 16 Fr. or 18 Fr. catheter, usually coudé tipped. The clinician places the prosthesis for the patient. If the patient's voice improves, he or she is instructed about the differences between the two prostheses in the following manner:

1. The differences in the tips and the lengths of the tips are explained.
2. The opening action of the conventional duckbill is compared with the recessed flap of the low-pressure voice prosthesis.
3. Attention is drawn to the fact that the very small ledge of the Baxter V. Mueller low-pressure voice prosthesis must be inserted carefully into the fistula with a slight upward push so that lateral and downward movement into the trachea is avoided.

In the early stages of using the low-pressure voice prosthesis, if the previously used duckbill-type prosthesis fits snugly, a low-pressure voice prosthesis that is one size longer might be used to ensure placement in the esophagus. Inserting the low-pressure voice prosthesis takes practice and must be closely monitored by the clinician.

No matter what type of patient you are working with, we strongly recommend the slow and easy approach to teaching prosthesis management. Our patients are frequently tense and anxious. The slow, easy approach pays dividends in the long run because the patient becomes more comfortable with the situation, the fistula, and the voice prosthesis.

Speech Pathologist's Time Commitments

In our experience, the number of visits per patient from insufflation to independent care and maintenance of the voice prosthesis varies widely. Therapy sessions range from 8 to 19, with the average being 12 30-min sessions per patient.

Costs

At $60 per session, the average cost of speech therapy is $738. If the actual therapy charge is coupled with the required materials, the total is approximately $1,000. This cost does not include the hospital, surgery, or operating room charges, which vary widely from one facility to another. The $1,000 estimate also does not include the cost of the tracheostoma speaking valve kit, or the cost of the clinic visits to determine the optimal valve diaphragm for the patient. Our patients prefer that we issue them the kit and bill the insurance carrier directly. With the hospital markup, the charge usually is $200 for the kit and $60 for the fitting session. The percentage of markup on the kit can be as much as 100% if the frequency of usage is low.

Insurance Coverage

We have experienced no difficulty in obtaining third-party coverage for pre- and postoperative TEP voice-restoration services. We have had patients from a variety of coverage plans, ranging from no insurance to Medicare, Blue Cross Blue Shield, Kaiser, as well as various preferred provider plans. Obviously, the surgical nature of the TEP procedure facilitates coverage of our required follow-up services.

TRACHEOSTOMA VALVE

Prior to having a patient try a tracheostoma valve, we require that he or she be able to speak effectively with manual stoma occlusion. Once the patient has learned manual occlusion, he or she is accustomed to the breathing and timing of speech and has gained insight into the inhalation and exhalation aspects of neck breathing.

When fitting the patient with the tracheostoma valve, we generally adhere to the following procedures. Initially, we ensure that the voice prosthesis is functioning properly. Next, we shorten the voice prosthesis strap approximately ¼ in. to allow the valve housing to cover it and prevent air leakage during speech. The exact length to cut off can be determined by placing the valve housing over the stoma and marking the place to cut on the strap. We strongly recommend cutting the strap after the prosthesis has been removed from the fistula to prevent the cut portion from being aspirated.

Preparation

We clean the area around the stoma with an alcohol swab. We are particularly cautious to wear gloves when working with voice prosthesis patients to avoid potential patient or clinician contamination. Although gloves become a hindrance when attempting to use the adhesive tape or the double-backed tape discs, they are still recommended.

After the stoma area has been cleaned with the alcohol, liquid adhesive is lightly applied around the patient's stoma. We use an inward–outward pattern, and have the patient observe in a mirror while we apply the adhesive. An outward pattern is used to preclude inadvertent dripping of the liquid adhesive into the stoma. We use disposable cotton-tipped swabs for this application since we often use a common bottle for different patients. We ensure that the adhesive is behind the voice prosthesis strap as well as over the top to avoid potential air leakage or blow-out problems.

While the adhesive is setting up, we demonstrate the mounting of the double-backed tape onto the tracheostoma valve housing. We have utilized Bivona tape, Baxter V. Mueller tape, Uro-Care foam discs, and the new Baxter V. Mueller heavy-duty tape discs (see the appendix for a list of supply sources). Some patients prefer one brand over another. Our own preference in the initial stages is to use the tracho-foam from Uro-Care because it is cushioned and is more easily fitted over the contours of the patient's neck. We have found that the regular Bivona and Baxter V. Mueller transparent double-backed tape tends to wrinkle when putting it on the valve housing. The tracho-foam disc is easily placed and air bubbles never form under it; however, it is very sticky and the adhesive substance is more difficult to remove from the valve housing once used. These discs also are more expensive than other products, costing $10 for a box of 30.

We have found that the new Baxter V. Mueller heavy-duty tape discs do not wrinkle as do the original transparent tape discs made by Bivona and Baxter V. Mueller. Our patients have reported that these new heavy-

duty tape discs stay on free of leaks for much longer periods of time than
do the older transparent tape discs. These new heavy-duty discs are also
much cheaper than are the foam-type discs.

When the liquid adhesive has set up around the patient's stoma, we
caution him or her to breathe easily to prevent coughing. Tracheal secretions on the adhesive will ruin the contact and result in an inadequate
seal. We have had patients who reflexively placed a tissue over their
stoma as they began to feel a cough sensation, which results in a coat
of white tissue paper stuck to the adhesive. This of course requires complete removal of the adhesive, followed by reapplication.

Placement

When the adhesive has dried we very carefully mount the tracheostoma
valve housing, trying to place the opening of the housing 1 or 2 mm
below the lower edge of the patient's stoma. We do this to provide a
natural trough for any mucus that comes from the stoma.

With patients who have had a narrow field laryngectomy, we find
it necessary to spread apart the sternocleidomastoids while we bend the
valve housing gently prior to placement. Generally, the one-handed
approach is used, with the forefinger guiding the opening of the valve
housing to the inferior border of the stoma and the thumb and middle
finger gently bending the valve housing outward as it approaches the
stoma.

Selecting the Optimal Diaphragm

Once the valve housing is over the stoma, one should firmly rub around
it, especially at the inward aspect near the opening. This can be done
very effectively with the blunt end of forceps or tweezers. After the valve
housing is in place, we usually start with an ultralight diaphragm made
by Baxter V. Mueller or Bivona. We explain to the patient that he or
she should breathe normally. We tell the patient that to activate the
diaphragm he or she must utilize a short inhalation followed by a quick
outward kind of exhalation to close it. The patient is then instructed
to follow these instructions and say /a/. Invariably patients will miss
a few initiations and the diaphragm will not close. Some will breathe
out too hard and close the valve for a longer phonation time than they
anticipate. When this occurs the clinician removes the tracheostoma
valve manually, allowing the back pressure of air to escape from behind
the valve. The patient is shown that he or she can remove the valve
at any time, but to be careful to remove it sideways, gently bending
upward while holding down the valve housing against the skin with
a finger to preclude any dislodgement of the housing's adhesive tape.

The patient is reminded not to grip the tracheostoma valve by the "bar" since it is designed specifically to hold clothing away from the valve, and is not sturdy enough to use when removing the valve.

The same steps essentially are used when having the patient try the Bivona Tracheostoma Valve II. The 15-g spring of the Tracheostoma Valve II corresponds to the ultralight diaphragm-type tracheostoma valve. The Bivona Tracheostoma Valve II does not have the "bar" in its design.

For practice we have the patient place the tracheostoma valve housing on a flat surface such as a mirror and then place the tracheostoma valve into the valve housing. Although the mirror provides a rigid surface, it is still a good approximation of what the patient will be working with on his or her own neck. Once the patient has learned how to insert the respiratory valve while looking at the mirror and valve housing, we then have him or her insert it without visual cues. The patient now acts as if the mirror is his or her neck and, without being able to see it, mounts the tracheostoma valve in the valve housing.

Another technique we have found beneficial is to have the patient mount the tracheostoma valve housing in the palm of his or her hand. Since this is soft tissue, it more closely approximates the patient's neck, and the patient can feel the sensation of pressure and misplacement of the valve while practicing with it.

When the patient is able to close the valve effectively for speech, we take a short walk around the clinic to see whether regular walking and breathing inadvertently activates spontaneous closure of the valve diaphragm or spring. The patient is required to walk briskly and sometimes go up a flight of stairs. If the ultralight diaphragm or 15-g spring is activated, we try a stiffer light diaphragm or heavier 20-g spring. We are interested in selecting a valve sensitivity that closes easily for speech but not during routine physical activity. Patients often are out of shape and brisk walking causes them to breathe slightly heavier than usual. This does not necessarily mean that they have the strength, timing, and respiratory capacity to activate the light diaphragm or the 20-g spring. Ninety percent of the patients we have worked with require an ultralight diaphragm or, in the case of the Tracheostoma Vent II, a 15-g spring with the lowest tension possible.

Advantages/Disadvantages

The Bivona Tracheostoma Vent II has many parts and requires cleaning and reassembling. Although it works well for some patients, older patients do not usually want something that comes apart and requires great dexterity for care and maintenance. Several of our patients have lost the tension springs from their Tracheostoma Vent II. Unfortunately, this renders the device inoperable.

Interestingly, 75% of the patients we treat do not use a tracheostoma speaking valve because they consider it too much trouble, or it will not adhere for long periods of time. Many are willing to use manual occlusion perhaps because they are not professional speakers, salespeople, or actively involved in social activities requiring hands-free speech. Our patients who use the tracheostoma valve include a retired auto dealer who did not like the idea of using his finger to occlude the stoma and wants to look as natural as possible in social situations, a retired businessman who plays golf and cards, a man who drives a motorcycle and talks a great deal on citizens band radio, a minister, and a supervisor at a textile factory. Several other patients who have the speaking valve use it periodically for social activities such as family or church gatherings. Eighty percent of our patients utilize a duckbill-type voice prosthesis and occlude their stomas with their thumb, middle, or index fingers. Some of our patients have large stomas and require the use of the tracheostoma valve housing to enable them to occlude their stomas with a finger. One of these, a woman, also has a modified insufflation test adapter attached to the valve housing to enable her to use her finger instead of her thumb.

Associated Problems

Problems that patients experience utilizing the tracheostoma valve housing are usually caused by the following:

- Failure to clean the skin around the stoma area adequately before attempting to gain adhesion.
- Less than optimal application of the liquid adhesive around the stoma, particularly in crevices, depressions, irregular contour areas, and/or around the prosthesis flap.
- Inappropriate mounting of the double-backed tape on the valve housing with some wrinkling of the tape.
- Transfer of oil from fingers to the sticky surface of the double-backed tape which reduces adhesion of the tape.
- Inadvertent coughing of mucus onto newly placed adhesive which reduces the effectiveness of the adhesion.
- Placement of the valve housing with outer edges adhering before optimal contact can be made with the inner aspect of the valve housing around the stoma.
- Placement of the valve housing too high relative to the stoma so that back-pressure and/or mucus can begin to erode the adhesive on the lower edge of the disc that is in contact with the patient's skin.

- Malpositioning of the valve housing which prevents good adhesion all around the stoma and promotes early blowout or leakage due to the small contact area.
- Failure of the patient to cover the complete voice prosthesis strap by at least 1 cm which allows escape of air and ultimate blowout of the valve housing.
- Removal of the tracheostoma valve with one hand which causes a strain on the adhesive of the valve housing and ultimately weakens it. The result is premature leakage and/or blowout.

Some patients attempt to compensate for air leakage by staggering tape in a circular fashion around the valve housing to ensure that the mounting stays in place. Other patients have success using only adhesive on the disc against the skin. Such patients do not use the double-backed tape disc. Usually these patients exert little strain on the valve housing because they have low back pressures.[1]

Measurement of Back Pressure

This measurement is most easily achieved by using the adapter from the Baxter V. Mueller auto-insufflation test set and coupling it to the manometer. In this manner the pressures can be read directly from the manometer during speech as the stoma is occluded. This is important because one common problem of seal breakdown is overinflation creating high back pressure. The patient can practice modifying his or her own back pressure by using the visual feedback from the manometer. The patient can begin to modify back pressure systematically toward a targeted lower pressure. Ultimately, it is desirable to activate and sustain tracheoesophageal puncture speech at a pressure of 40 cm/H_2O or less.

NEW DEVELOPMENTS

A number of new developments are in progress or currently on the market. These are aimed at alleviating some of the problems experienced by patients who have undergone tracheoesophageal puncture. Recently, Blom and Singer have addressed the difficulty with air leaks around the tracheostoma valve housing. They have introduced a more aggressive tape disc manufactured by Baxter V. Mueller. These tape discs have proven to last considerably longer than the original double-backed tape discs that are marketed by Bivona and Baxter V. Mueller.

---

1. James Liedman (1989) described success in using only Skin Prep instead of silicone adhesives for adhering the valve housing to the peristomal area. This product is available from United Medical, Largo, FL.

Another type of double-backed tape disc manufactured by Uro-Care is the tracho-foam disc (product 5300). Although this is not a new development, it is a type of disc with which many speech–language pathologists may not be familiar. It has proven useful with certain patients whose stomal and/or neck configurations require a more flexible and contour-shaped double-backed disc.

Most recently Barton, DeSanto, Pearson, and Keith (1988) reported their development of an endostomal tracheostomy tube for leakproof retention of the Blom-Singer tracheostoma valve. The appliance consists of a soft silicone rubber collar measuring $8 \times 27 \times 3$ mm. Reportedly, it will accept any tracheostoma valve currently being manufactured. Presently the button is available only through the Mayo Clinic Engineering Department, but plans are to market it soon through the Baxter V. Mueller Company.

The pharyngeal plexus neurectomy described initially by Singer el al. (1986) seems to be supplanting the inferior constrictor myotomy procedure. More surgeons are beginning to perform a pharyngeal plexus neurectomy at the time of primary laryngectomy. Ultimately, this may result in fewer myotomies being performed at the time of TEP.

In November 1988, Bivona announced the availability of their Ultra low resistance voice prosthesis in both 20 Fr. and 16 Fr. sizes. The low resistance of the 20 Fr. size promises to be beneficial to selected patients.

One persistent and always potential problem is an inadvertent closure of the fistula due to dislodgement of the voice prosthesis. This results in patients having to undergo repuncture, which is inconvenient and costly. E. D. Blom and M. I. Singer (personal communication, June 4, 1988) are currently in the final stages of development and clinical evaluation of a permanent in-dwelling stent. This device is designed to remain in the patient's fistula and prevent closure. Reportedly, a Baxter V. Mueller voice prosthesis of the appropriate size will be easily removed and reinserted within this stent. This type of in-dwelling stent will preclude having to dilate the patient with catheters because the stent will maintain the shape of the fistula tract.

APPENDIX

Item	Description	Use
Urological Catheters	#14 Regular tip	Preop air insufflation testing.
	#12 Regular tip	Postop backup for emergency.
	#14 Coudé tip	Postop safety, kept in fistula while cleaning stoma or voice prosthesis.
	#16 Coudé tip	Postop, used to dilate fistula slightly for regular voice prosthesis.
	#18 Coudé tip	Postop, used to dilate fistula for placement of Blom–Singer low-pressure voice prosthesis.
	#20 Coudé tip	Postop, used to dilate fistula after use of #16 and #18, to dilate fistula further for insertion of Bivona low-resistance voice prosthesis.
	#10 Regular tip (with tip cut off)	Postop, used to troubleshoot and/or check function of TEP by placing within voice prostheses and insufflating. Facilitates testing without requiring stoma occlusion.
	#14 Foley with 5-cc balloon	Placed intraoperatively to maintain TE fistula. The myotomized patient can also be fed via this tube, thus precluding the placement of a nasogastric tube for feeding.

Manufacturer: BARD Urological Division, C. R. Bard, Inc., Murray Hill, NJ 07974

Rubber Gloves		Working around patient's stoma, in contact with tracheal secretions and/or blood. Prevents clinician-to-patient contamination and/or patient-to-clinician contamination.

Manufacturer: Beckton Dickinson, Tru-Touch Gloves (small, medium, large)

Item	Description	Use
Blom-Singer	Individual auto-insufflation kits complete with tape discs; standardized, marked catheter and connector; and specific instructions for mounting and use	To enable the patient to use the pulmonary support system to activate esophageal phonation in an attempt to approximate the postop system.

Manufacturer: Baxter Healthcare Corporation, 1500 Waukegan Rd., McGaw Park, IL 60085

Item	Description	Use
Suture Removal Set	Tweezers, curved	Stoma care.
	Forceps	Gripping prosthetic flap.
	Scissors	Releasing catheter postop when necessary.
	(Sterilized between patients)	

Manufacturer: Usually obtained from otolaryngologist

Item	Description	Use
Viscous Lidocaine	2% viscous lidocaine hydrochloride oral topical solution	Lubrication of catheters and prostheses, when necessary with some patients.
Saline Solution	.09% sodium chloride irrigation solution	Flushing sticky voice prostheses by placing tip of eye dropper full of saline into front opening of voice prostheses.
Eyedropper	Standard medical eyedropper	

Manufacturer: Travenol Laboratories, Inc., Deerfield, IL

Item	Description	Use
Cotton Swabs	Long, wooden-handled type	Placing valve housing adhesive, removal of stomal tracheal secretions near stoma.
Tape	1 in., hypoallergenic	To maintain position of prosthesis flap.
Alcohol Packets	Standard, individually wrapped alcohol pads	To clean stomal area prior to adhesive application.

Manufacturer: The Clinipad Corporation, Guilford, CT

Adhesive Removal Wipes	Unisolve adhesive removal wipes, 50/box	Removal of tracheostoma speaking valve adhesive.

Manufacturer: Unisolve, Division of Howell Medical, Inc., 11775 Starkey Rd., Largo, FL 33543

Voice Prostheses Regular Type	Blom-Singer voice prostheses, Sizes 1.8, 2.2, 2.6, 3.0, 3.3, and 3.6 cm	Fitting of patients. Should have enough of each to provide patient with at least one backup. Stock many more of the shorter sizes than the longer sizes.
Low Pressure	1.8, 2.2, 2.6, 3.0, 3.3, and 3.6 cm	
Sizing Device	Calibrated sizer	To determine proper length of prosthesis to be inserted postoperatively.
Tracheostoma Speaking Valves	Professional fitting kit, complete with different diaphragms (ultralight, light, medium) or springs (15, 20, 25, and 30 ga)	
Tape Disks		Used to mount valve housing.

Item	Description	Use
Valve Housings		Mounted over stoma to hold tracheostoma speaking valves.
Heavy Duty Tape Disks*		Stronger tape designed to last longer and reduce possibility of leaks or blowouts of valve housings.

Manufacturers: Baxter V. Mueller, American Hospital Supply Corp.,
6600 West Touhy Ave., Chicago, IL 60648-4588
and
Bivona, Inc., 5700 West 23rd. Ave., Gary, IN 46406
*Baxter V. Mueller only

Item	Description	Use
Suction Device 561	Built-in or portable suction device with removable tubing which can extend to patient's stoma and tracheal areas, preferably with sterile, stainless suction	Very useful at initial postop sessions when patient is more likely to cough, swallow, and/or regurgitate reflexively.

Manufacturer: DeVilbiss Co., Somerset, PA 15501

REFERENCES

Amatsu, M., Matsui, T., Maki, T., & Kanagawa, K. (1977). Vocal reconstruction after total laryngectomy: A new one-stage surgical technique. *Journal of Otolaryngology (Japan), 80,* 779–785.

Andrews, J. C., Mickel, R. A., Hanson, D. G., Monahan, G. P., & Ward, P. H. (1987). Major complications following tracheo-esophageal puncture for voice rehabilitation. *Laryngoscope, 97,* 562–567.

Asai, R. (1972). Laryngoplasty after total laryngectomy. *Archives of Otolaryngology, 95,* 114.

Barton, D., DeSanto, L., Pearson, B. W., & Keith, R. (1988). An endostomal tracheostomy tube for leakproof retention of the Blom-Singer stomal valve. *Otolaryngology, Head and Neck Surgery, 99,* 38–41.

Blom, E. D., & Singer, M. I. (1979). Surgical–prosthetic approaches for postlaryngectomy voice restoration. In R. L. Keith & F. Darley (Eds.), *Laryngectomy rehabilitation* (pp. 251–276). Austin, TX: PRO-ED.

Blom, E. D., Singer, M. I., & Hamaker, R. C. (1981). Further experience with voice restoration after total laryngectomy. *Annals of Otolaryngology, 90,* 498–502.

Blom, E. D., Singer, M. I., & Hamaker, R. C. (1985). An improved esophageal insufflation test. *Archives of Otolaryngology, 111,* 211–212.

Conley, J. J., DeAmesti, F., & Pierce, J. K. (1958). A new surgical technique for the vocal rehabilitation of the laryngectomized patient. *Annals of Otology, Rhinology and Laryngology, 67,* 655–664.

Damsté, P. H. (1958). *Oesophageal speech after laryngectomy.* Groningen, The Netherlands: Gebroeders Hoitsema.

Diedrich, W. M. (1968). The mechanism of esophageal speech. In A. Bouhuys (Ed.), *Sound production in man* (Vol. 155, pp. 303–320). New York: The Academy.

Hamaker, R. C., Singer, M. I., & Blom, E. D. (1985). Primary voice restoration at laryngectomy. *Archives of Otolaryngology, 111,* 182–186.

Hudgins, C. V., Hawkins, J. E., Karlin, J. E., & Stevens, S. S. (1947). The development of recorded auditory tests for measuring hearing loss for speech. *Laryngoscope, 57,* 57–89.

Keith, R. L., Shane, H. C., Coates, H. L. C., & Devine, K. D. (1984). *Looking forward: A guidebook for the laryngectomee.* New York: Thieme-Stratton.

Liedman, J. A. (1989). *Overview of laryngectomee rehabilitation.* Paper presented at the 1989 State Annual Meeting of Laryngectomees, Williamsburg, VA.

Moon, J. D., & Weinberg, B. (1987). Aerodynamic and myoelastic contributions to tracheo-esophageal voice production. *Journal of Speech and Hearing Research, 30,* 387–395.

Robbins, J. A. (1984). Acoustic differentiation of laryngeal, esophageal, and tracheoesophageal speech. *Journal of Speech and Hearing Research, 27,* 577–585.

Robbins, J. A., Fisher, H. B., Blom, E. D., & Singer, M. I. (1984). A comparative acoustic study of normal, esophageal, and tracheo-esophageal speech production. *Journal of Speech and Hearing Disorders, 49,* 202–210.

Rubin, H. (1959). *High speed cinematography of the pathologic larynx* [Film]. Los Angeles: Cedars of Lebanon Hospital.

Schuller, D. E., Jarrow, J. E., Kelly, D. R., & Miglets, A. W. (1983). Prognostic factors affecting the success of duckbill vocal restoration. *Otolaryngology, Head and Neck Surgery, 91,* 396–398.

Singer, M. I., & Blom, E. D. (1978). *Presentation of preliminary results with the tracheoesophageal fistula technique of Amatsu.* Paper presented at Second International Workshop of the Surgical and Prosthetic Speech Rehabilitation Study Group, Buffalo, New York.

Singer, M. I., & Blom, E. D. (1980). An endoscopic technique for restoration of voice after laryngectomy. *Annals of Otology, Rhinology and Laryngology, 89,* 529–533.

Singer, M. I., Blom, E. D., & Hamaker, R. C. (1986). Pharyngeal plexus neurectomy for alaryngeal speech rehabilitation. *Laryngoscope, 96,* 50–53.

Sisson, G. A., Bytell, D. E., Becker, S. P., McConnel, F. M. S., & Singer, M. I. (1978). Total laryngectomy and reconstruction of a pseudoglottis: Problems and complications. *Laryngoscope, 88,* 639–650.

Taub, S., & Spiro, R. H. (1972). Vocal rehabilitation of laryngectomees: Preliminary report of a new technique. *American Journal of Surgery, 124,* 87–90.

Van den Berg, J., & Moolenaar-Bijl, A. J. (1959). Cricopharyngeal sphincter, pitch, intensity, and fluency in oesophageal speech. *Practica Oto-rhino-laryngologica, 21,* 298–315.

Wetmore, S. J., Johns, M. E., & Baker, S. R. (1981). The Singer–Blom voice restoration procedure. *Archives of Otolaryngology, 107,* 674–676.

Wetmore, S. J., Krueger, K., Wesson, K., & Blessing, M. L. (1985). Long term results of the Blom–Singer speech rehabilitation procedure. *Archives of Otolaryngology, 111,* 106–109.

CHAPTER 7

Treatment Following Tracheoesophageal Fistulization Surgery

Zilpha T. Bosone

Bosone presents a step-by-step procedure for the inexperienced clinician to follow when initiating a clinical program with patients having undergone tracheoesophageal fistulization surgery. Her attention to detail in the problem-solving section of the chapter will be of interest to even the most experienced. Self-care responsibilities are discussed. The materials patients need to function independently also are delineated.

Study Questions

1. In addition to length, what are at least six ways in which voice prostheses may differ structurally?
2. What are three potential advantages for extending the time the catheter is left in the fistula after surgery?
3. There is a hierarchy for making sound. What are three ways of potentially activating the sound generator, proceeding from the simplest to the most complex?
4. How does one differentially diagnose leaking through the prosthesis from leaking around the prosthesis?

INITIAL CLINIC SUPPLIES

To begin treating patients who have had tracheosophageal fistula (TEF) procedures for voice restoration after laryngectomy, the clinician needs to have on hand some basic supplies. Determining what constitutes "basic supplies" is not a simple matter, however, because the variety of prostheses and related equipment grows larger each year.

Prostheses

The clinician needs to consider quantity, size, and style when thinking about which prostheses to order. The quantity is determined by whether one is going to issue or sell prostheses directly to patients, or whether the prostheses on hand will be used only for trial fittings. It is less encumbering to do the latter. Once the appropriate style and length of prosthesis has been decided for a patient, he or she may use the "loaner" until the new prosthesis arrives, or keep the "loaner" and donate a new one to the clinician, or be stented with a catheter, the outside diameter of which is compatible with the new prosthesis. The most common prosthesis lengths seem to be 2.2 and 2.6 cm. Shorter and longer sizes are available from the regular stock of most suppliers, and some companies will even custom-make a prosthesis to fit specifications. Although prostheses come in a variety of styles, not all styles need to be represented in a clinician's basic supply. The following list contains suggested sizes and quantities from the two major suppliers. When a new prosthesis comes on the market, the clinician should test it on a few selected patients before purchasing a supply in all sizes.

Bivona Surgical, Inc.		Baxter V. Mueller	
Size (in cm)	Quantity	Size (in cm)	Quantity
16 Fr. with collar		16 Fr. Blom–Singer	
2.2	4–6	1.8	2
2.6	4–6	2.2	2
3.0	2	2.6	2
3.3	1	3.0	1
3.6	1		
20 Fr. low-resistance		16 Fr. low-pressure	
2.2	2	2.2	2
2.6	2	2.6	2
3.0	1	3.0	1

The rationale for selecting these four prosthesis styles is presented in the section on prostheses that follows.

Sizing Devices

Sizing devices need to be part of the basic supplies. Two Bivona sizing devices in 16 Fr. and one in 20 Fr., all with retention collars, are recommended for use in determining what prosthesis size matches the length of the fistula. Although other companies make sizing devices, the Bivona is recommended because the soft retention collar allows easy insertion and withdrawal.

Catheters

All-purpose catheters have many uses before, during, and after TEF surgery. It is advisable to keep a good supply on hand at all times. If buying in small quantities of less than 100, call medical supply houses for the best price. The cost per catheter can range from $1.50 to $5. If buying in boxes of 100, the cost is around $45/box. The catheters are identified as general purpose or all purpose, and are 16 in. long. The red rubber catheters are softer and more pliable than the orange, or "Rob-Nel," catheters. The red rubber catheters can be purchased from Davol Inc. and the Inmed Corp., among others. The less pliable, more penetrating Rob-Nel catheters are available from the Argyle Division of Sherwood Medical Industries, for example. The Rob-Nel catheters are useful in opening fistulas that have stenosed or closed. The following sizes and quantities are suggested:

- 10 each red rubber in sizes 20 Fr., 16 Fr., and 14 Fr.
- 10 each Rob-Nel in sizes 20 Fr., 18 Fr., 16 Fr., and 14 Fr.
- 20 each Rob-Nel in sizes 12 Fr. and 10 Fr.

Tracheostoma Valve Fitting Kit

Tracheostoma valve professional fitting kits are available from Bivona and Baxter V. Mueller. Both are essentially the same. Only one kit is needed, and the final selection is a matter of personal preference.

Back Pressure Gauge/Manometer

The clinician can make a device for measuring back pressure after a tracheoesophageal fistulization procedure. In this case, back pressure is the pressure of the air that will be pushing against the finger or tracheostoma valve when the patient is speaking. If this pressure is too high, it can loosen the housing of a tracheostoma valve and eventually cause a leak. The original suggestion for making and using the pressure-measuring device was given to me by Eric Blom (personal conversation, July 28, 1986). The following parts are needed: (a) a pressure gauge or manometer that measures up to at least 60 cm of water; (b) the catheter and white tracheostoma adapter from a Blom–Singer Esophageal Insufflation Test Set (available from Baxter V. Mueller); (c) a 16 Fr. Rob-Nel general-purpose catheter, or any catheter having an internal diameter that will allow a good flow of air, and whose ends are compatible with the fittings on the gauge and tracheostoma adapter; and (d) a tracheostoma valve housing. To construct the device, attach one end of the catheter to the tracheostoma adapter, and the other end to the pressure gauge. If the catheter already attached to the tracheostoma adapter is too small to go over the fitting on the pressure gauge, the 16 Fr. Rob-Nel may be substituted. To do this, remove the adapter and attach it to the small end of the catheter, which has been cut to expose the lumen. Then attach the large, tapered end to the pressure gauge.

To use the pressure gauge, affix the tracheostoma valve housing to the peristomal area, following the directions given with the Blom–Singer Esophageal Insufflation Test Set, or with the tracheostoma valve kit. Insert the large end of the tracheostoma adapter into the housing. Either the patient or the clinician can occlude the open end of the adapter with a finger, and the clinician watches the gauge as the patient uses conversational speech. Blom advised that pressures during speaking should not exceed 40 cm H_2O. Higher pressures can break the seal of the housing. If the patient exceeds this value, the gauge can be used therapeutically to provide feedback to the user as one means of attempting to lower back pressure.

Additional Items

Additional items to complete the list of basic supplies include:

1-in. paper tape	1 box
Gauze sponges, 4 × 4, not sterile	1 package
Forceps, 6 in. thumb	2 each
Cotton-tipped applicators, 6 in.	1 package of 100
Water soluble lubricant	1 tube
Pipe cleaners	3 packages
Scissors	1 pair
Green or blue food coloring	1 bottle

USE OF CATHETERS

All-purpose catheters are used before, during, and after TEF surgery. Before surgery, they can be used for the esophageal insufflation test. If the surgical procedure is a Singer–Blom type, a catheter is positioned in the fistula to keep the fistula open, and to prevent food or liquid from entering the airway during healing. Catheters, especially the Rob-Nel, more rigid type, can be used to reopen a fistula that is stenosed or has recently closed. Catheters can be used as temporary replacements for the prosthesis, for example, when the prosthesis is being cleaned, or when the prosthesis leaks or otherwise fails to function properly. When the fistula must be enlarged to use a larger diameter prosthesis, the fistula is up-stented by using a larger diameter catheter prior to insertion of the prosthesis. When the diameter of the fistula must be reduced to accept a smaller prosthesis, or as part of reversing the procedure (letting the fistula close), down-stenting is done with smaller diameter catheters until the desired size is reached.

At Time of Surgery

At the time of surgery, the catheter placed in the fistula to keep it open and prevent aspiration is usually 14 Fr. in diameter. It is advantageous to have the catheter directed downward in the esophagus rather than upward and exiting from the mouth or nose. The downward position is far more comfortable for the patient, especially if it is to be left in for several days. When the fistula has been stented upward, the tendency is to fit with a prosthesis that is too long, and therefore maintains the upward direction of the fistula. In addition, when this situation occurs, the tracheal end of the prosthesis is tilted downward into the stoma and is consequently likely to catch more discharge. When the catheter is directed down the esophagus, the prosthesis is easier to fit, and it seems to rest immediately in the ideal horizontal position.

The distal tip of the catheter can be directed downward in the esophagus at the time of surgery. Alternatively, if the catheter has been directed through the nose or mouth, the following simple procedure can be used to position it downward. A day or two after surgery, a new catheter is prepared by threading a guide wire through it to the distal tip. The distal end is then bent to a gentle downward curve. If the new catheter were to be inserted into the fistula without the addition of the curve, it would follow the course of the original fistula and move upward toward the mouth. The original catheter is withdrawn, and the new wired catheter is inserted into the fistula with the curve going downward. As the tip enters the esophagus, in about 2–3 cm, the guide wire is gradually withdrawn as the catheter is advanced. When the guide wire is out and the catheter is in place, a knot is tied near the end of the catheter to prevent reflux, and it is taped to the side of the neck. The 14 Fr. catheter is tolerated well; in fact, patients usually forget its presence. If the patient requires a larger fistula lumen to be compatible with the prosthesis, it can be done by up-stenting from 3 hr to overnight prior to fitting the prosthesis.

Extended Duration of Stenting After Surgery

The catheter is commonly left in for about 48 hr prior to fitting a prosthesis. There are, however, advantages for extending this period to a minimum of 10 days. One advantage is that extending stenting allows more time for the fistula to heal, thereby reducing the edema and increasing the chances that the prosthesis size will be suitable for a longer time. It is often necessary to reduce the length of the prosthesis as time passes, but when the patient is fit after 48 hr, more frequent changes may be necessary. While the catheter is in place, routine hygiene continues. The tape is removed, the peristomal area is thoroughly cleaned, and new taping is done. Another advantage of extending the healing time is that more prostheses have a retention collar, which is a flange that rests against the esophageal wall, and is larger in diameter than the body of the prosthesis. It can be abrasive to a newly formed fistula, and cause bleeding and discomfort when measuring devices and prostheses, also with retention collars, are inserted and withdrawn by the clinician and patient during sessions for fitting and prosthesis management training.

Extended stenting has the major benefit of providing the opportunity for the patient to develop some proficiency with TEF speech by removing the catheter and phonating via the open fistula. Tracheal air flows with less resistance through the open fistula than through the prosthesis. Shagets and Panje (1985) suggested that patients remove the catheter and practice vocalization four to six times a day for 15- to 30-min intervals until relaxed proficiency is achieved, usually within 2–4 weeks. While the catheter is out, the patient is cautioned not to swallow because of the risk of aspiration. The prosthesis is inserted after satisfactory speech is achieved with the open fistula.

PROSTHESES

This section describes characteristics of the current prostheses from the two major suppliers and provides rationales for choices.

Retention Collars

Bivona still makes the original prosthesis which has no retention collar. It comes in diameters of 16 and 20 Fr. Although prostheses with retention collars are most frequently used, some consumers continue to use the original style. Prostheses without retention collars should be selected only if the fistula tract is 3.3 cm or longer, and the patient does not have hard or frequent coughing. In addition, the patient must be able to manage the more extensive taping procedures that are necessary to retain the original type of prosthesis in place.

Most prostheses have retention collars, which reduce the possibility of accidental dislodging. This is especially important when the patient coughs frequently, when the fistula track is short, or when a significant portion of the prosthesis is unsupported by the fistula track. The latter may occur when the back wall of the trachea is deep in relation to the stoma. Prostheses with retention collars are made by Bivona in diameters of 16 and 20 Fr., and by Baxter V. Mueller (Blom–Singer) in 16 Fr. Bivona makes two styles of retention collars. The lightweight, small-diameter collar on their duckbill and low-resistance voice prostheses offers little resistance on insertion and withdrawal, yet is effective in maintaining the prosthesis in place. The Bivona Economy Duckbill Prosthesis and all Blom–Singer prostheses have a significantly stiffer, larger diameter retention collar, requiring up-stenting with an 18 Fr. catheter prior to inserting. These prostheses are especially useful if the patient has difficulty retaining those with more delicate retention collars.

Resistance to Airflow

Low-resistance/low-pressure prostheses may be beneficial in those cases in which the resistance of other prostheses interferes with optimum sound production. This interference possibility may be tested by comparing the patient's ease of sound production using the open fistula and then the prosthesis. If sound production is less effortful with the open fistula, the patient may benefit by changing to a prosthesis with reduced resistance to airflow. Bivona offers a 20 Fr. low-resistance prosthesis which as the least resistance to airflow of any prosthesis tested and reported in the literature (Smith, 1986; Weinberg & Moon, 1984, 1986a, 1986b).

Length of Esophageal End

The Blom–Singer 16 Fr. low-pressure prosthesis has the shortest esophageal end. Only 2 mm of the prosthesis extends into the lumen of the esophagus, whereas the Bivona low-resistance model and the duckbill designs from both companies extend 8 mm. A prosthesis with a shortened esophageal tip should be considered when irritation occurs from the esophageal end of an otherwise properly fitted prosthesis.

Ease of Insertion

Features other than the design of the retention collar, resistance to air-flow, and length of esophageal end of the prosthesis should also be considered. For example, ease of insertion of the prosthesis is determined by the shape of the esophageal end as well as the diameter and stiffness of the retention collar. The duckbill or "bullet-nosed" tip is easiest to insert. The relatively open ends on the Bivona low-resistance and Blom–Singer low-pressure prostheses offer considerably more resistance.

Neck Strap(s)

Bivona makes prostheses with two horizontal neck straps or, upon request, a single vertical strap. All Blom–Singer prostheses have one vertical strap. The vertical straps have the advantages of being easier to tape, less apt to catch tracheal discharge, and less interfering with finger occlusion of the stoma.

Opaqueness

Not all prostheses are radiopaque; that is, they cannot all be seen on X-ray should the prosthesis be aspirated. All Blom–Singer prostheses and the Bivona Economy Duckbill are radiopaque.

Combined with Tracheostoma Vent

The patient may need to use a laryngectomy tube or stoma vent in combination with a prosthesis because of stomal stenosis or megastoma. Bivona makes the Bivona–Colorado Voice Prosthesis, which combines a tracheostoma vent with any style and size Bivona prosthesis. Instead of the single unit, the prosthesis and stoma vent can be made compatible by inserting the prosthesis of choice, then inserting the stoma vent which has been selected according to appropriate length and diameter. The prosthesis should not have an air entry port on the inferior surface. The location of the prosthesis is visualized through the inside, superior surface of the stoma vent, and outlined with a marking pen. Blom (1989) suggests making a ⅛-in.-wide slit across the site of the center opening in the prosthesis. Another method is to cut a window in the stoma vent to match the location and diameter of the center opening of the prosthesis. The edges are buffed smooth to prevent irritation. Buffing equipment can be found in dental, prosthetic, or earmold laboratories. Robert L. Keith, of the Mayo Clinic (personal communication, December 29, 1988), suggests using emery boards with coarse and fine grain. One board of each grain is cut to fit within the lumen of the window. The edges of the window are buffed, using the coarse-grained board first, and finished with the fine-grained board. The stoma vent can then be inserted and the tracheal end of the prosthesis will protrude slightly from the window. Occlusion of the stoma vent will shunt air through the center opening of the prosthesis.

USING THE PROSTHESIS

Initial Session

The initial session combines fitting the prosthesis with producing sound. The patient will be given the opportunity to insert the prosthesis one or two times during the session, alternating insertions with speech attempts. The number of insertions and withdrawals of measuring devices and prostheses with retention collars should be kept to the minimum necessary to achieve the desired result; otherwise, irritation may cause some edema in the fistula and alter the measurements, as well as cause discomfort for the patient.

There is an hierarchy for making sound after TEF surgery. The easiest way for the patient to make sound is when the clinician inserts a 14 Fr. catheter into the fistula for a distance of about 4 cm, and blows a steady stream of air into the esophagus. This requires no effort on the part of the patient. The next, and slightly more difficult step in the hierarchy is to have the patient try to produce sound with the prosthesis removed. The patient or clinician can occlude the stoma with a finger as the patient exhales. The most difficult step is to produce sound with the prosthesis in place. Thus, the prosthesis should not be fit unless the patient can produce sound by the first two steps. If the patient has been stented with a catheter for a minimum of 10 days since surgery, and has been successfully producing sound with the catheter removed, there is a good possibility sound will be produced when the prosthesis is inserted.

Although most patients who are carefully selected for the TEF procedure are successful in making sound at the initial treatment session, some do not. The initial session has a highly emotional atmosphere. It is widely recognized that esophageal sound and emotionally charged situations are not always compatible. For this reason, and to lessen the tension somewhat, the patient should be told that he or she may not make sound during the first session. If there is difficulty at one step, the clinician may have to alternate between the previous step at which the patient made sound and the next level where the difficulty occurs. Syllables with initial /h/ are good for stimulating exhalation and sound production. If single syllables or words are not successful, automatic speech, sentences, or spontaneous conversation may relieve some of the stress and result in sound.

The prosthesis stimulates saliva flow, and the increase in the amount of saliva negatively influences articulation and sound resonance. The patient should be encouraged not only to swallow frequently, but to use the watery or muffled quality of the sound being produced as a cue to the need for additional swallows. After TEF surgery, the patient can produce effective throat clearing by closing the mouth, inhaling moderately, occluding the stoma, and exhaling a steady stream while making a long "hum-m-m" sound.

Behaviors Counterproductive to Sound Generation

Many behaviors are counterproductive to sound generation. One is breath holding when the stoma is occluded. Some patients are slow to get the idea that it is possible for them to exhale when the stoma is occluded; their first inclination is to hold their breath. To determine whether the patient is holding his or her breath, the clinician should occlude the stoma, ask the patient to produce sound, and as the attempt is being made, quickly release the occlusion and feel and listen for the escaping air which should be present if the patient is exhaling.

The patient will frequently inhale deeply and exhale forcefully in attempting sound production. This attempt may be associated with excessive effort, or with pushing for loud sound. Such behavior can cause an air leak around the occluded stoma, and the physical strain can either prevent sound or produce a sound that is too loud or too short. A decrease in depth and force of respiration may be brought about by encouraging the patient to think of whispering. The result will not be a whisper, but thinking in that vein should stimulate relaxation, reduced loudness, and easy exhalation.

The patient who used esophageal speech prior to the TEF surgery may try to retain the habit of air charging prior to initiation of sound. This behavior can usually be eliminated by having the patient hold open his or her mouth, and begin speech attempts with /ha/ as a starter.

OCCLUDING THE STOMA

To shunt lung air through the fistula and into the esophagus, exhaled air must not be allowed to escape through the stoma. The stoma is occluded by a finger or thumb, or by a tracheostoma valve. Occluding the stoma manually is not simple. One problem is pressing too hard on the stoma, which should be avoided by the clinician and the patient. Excessive pressure can narrow the lumen of the esophagus, restricting inflation, making the patient exert more energy, and effectively altering sound quality or cutting off sound completely. Too much pressure on the stoma may push the prosthesis deep into the fistula, which has two possible ramifications. The esophageal end of the prosthesis may impinge on the back wall of the esophagus so that airflow is restricted or completely blocked. Second, the air entry port, which is on the underside of many prostheses, may be occluded. This would not be a major concern if air could enter the prosthesis through the center opening; however, in some cases, the prosthesis protrudes so far anteriorly that manual occlusion of the stoma also covers the center opening of the prosthesis. Another consideration related to manual occlusion is that stoma noise and air wastage may result from (a) insufficient finger pressure, (b) a wet peristomal area, (c) use of a finger or thumb that is too small for complete occlusion, or (d) a stoma that is too large to cover manually.

Here are some guidelines for occluding the stoma. Manual occlusion should be complete, but gentle. The peristomal area must be kept clean and dry. The anterior portion of the neck, around and superior to the stoma, must be allowed to move forward on phonation. This is a natural occurrence when the esophagus inflates. The finger or thumb should ride the neck as it swells anteriorly, and not restrict this movement in any way. When the stoma is too large for the finger or thumb to make a good seal, one should consider using a stoma vent/prosthesis combination (see section entitled "Prostheses" for description). The flange on the stoma vent effectively seals the edges of the stoma when pressure is applied, and the vent itself has a smaller internal lumen than the stoma, making it easier to occlude manually.

Several decisions remain to be made regarding occlusions of the stoma. Should the dominant or nondominant hand be used? It is preferable to use the nondominant hand if the occlusion is good, and the hand can be positioned gracefully and subtly. Which finger or thumb should be used? Whichever one provides the best seal and allows the best posture. Should the occlusion be over or under the stoma cover? It is less cumbersome, less distracting, and faster if done over the stoma cover, but this is not always successful. Most people improve with practice. To obtain a satisfactory seal over the stoma cover, it may be necessary to experiment with various fabrics, materials, and combinations. On the other hand, some individuals either prefer to or have to go under the stoma cover. This is not a problem as long as it can be done with speed and minimal distraction. Is a tracheostoma valve a possibility? A tracheostoma valve is ideal if it can be worn all day without developing a leak in the housing. Wearing the valve eliminates all of the problems associated with manual occlusion, and allows the user to have both hands free.

IMPORTANT OBSERVATIONS AND THEIR IMPLICATIONS

Leaking

The patient may notice an increase in the amount of coughing or the presence of colored discharge on the stoma cover. The discharge may be the color of coffee, gelatin, or some other liquid recently swallowed. There are two possible sites for the leakage of swallowed material into the trachea: *around* the prosthesis and *through* the prosthesis. It is important to identify the site because the treatments are different.

The location of the leak can be determined by adding a few drops of dark food coloring to a glass of water. Remove most of the cotton from a 6-in. cotton-tipped applicator, leaving just enough cotton to allow passage of the applicator into the center opening of the prosthesis. With the prosthesis in place in the fistula, insert the swabbed end of the applicator into the center opening, and just beyond the air entry port on the under-surface of the prosthesis. An observer should be positioned to get a good view of the fistula, using a flashlight. The patient should take a small sip of the colored water and hold it in the mouth until told by the observer to swallow. At that point, the observer watches the fistula for any trace of colored water. If any is seen, it is leaking *around* the prosthesis. If none is seen, but when the applicator is withdrawn there is coloring on the cotton, the leak is *through* the prosthesis. This test may need to be repeated with larger amounts of colored water being swallowed.

If the leak is *around* the prosthesis, the implication is that the lumen of the fistula has enlarged and is no longer fitting snugly around the shaft of the prosthesis. This condition may develop spontaneously over time, or it may be due to wearing a prosthesis that is too long. When the prosthesis is too long, the act of swallowing may push down on the esophageal end, momentarily widening, and possibly eventually enlarging the diameter of the fistula. Solutions to this problem include using a shorter prosthesis, if appropriate, and using one with a retention collar. Retention collars not only reduce the possibility of accidentally dislodging the prosthesis, but also make a good seal around the esophageal end of the fistula during swallowing. One could also remove the prosthesis at night, and replace it with a catheter of a smaller diameter (e.g., a 12 Fr. catheter for a 16 Fr. prosthesis). If none of these suggestions is effective in stopping the leak, the otorhinolaryngologist may try electrocauterization (Singer & Blom, 1980; Singer, Blom, & Hamaker, 1981). In this procedure, a small charge of electrical current is applied to two or three spots inside of the fistula. This action contracts the tissues, and reduces the lumen of the fistula. One treatment is usually sufficient to achieve the desired result.

If the leak is *through* the prosthesis, the most likely cause is normal wear and tear. Most prostheses last a minimum of 2–3 months, and one may expect signs of leakage around that time. The solution is to replace the prosthesis. On the other hand, if the prosthesis leaks prematurely (and this can be after only a few days of use), it may be too long, or candida organisms may be attacking it. The prosthesis that is too long may leak because of abuse to the esophageal end during speech and swallowing. Again, a proper-fitting prosthesis is essential.

Candida.   The deterioration of silicone voice prostheses caused by the candida organism was first described by a group from the Netherlands (Mahieu, Rosingh, Saene, & Schutte, 1985). Subsequent articles have provided more detailed information and suggestions for treatment (Blom & Singer, 1986; Izdebski, Ross, & Lee, 1987; Mahieu, H. K. F. van Saene, Rosingh, & Schutte, 1986; Mahieu, J. J. M. van Saene, den Besten, & H. K. F. van Saene, 1986; Modica, 1987). The presence and quantity of candida organisms are determined by laboratory tests of a culture taken from the fistula and/or prosthesis. Candida is a yeast that is part of the normal oral flora. Its existence in increased quantities is common in cancer patients. Chemotherapy and radiation therapy are listed among other factors that promote favorable environments for fungal growth (Rodu, Griffin, & Gockerman, 1984). The organism seems to have a "high affinity for silicone, resulting in adherence, cleaving, and invasive growth" into the prosthesis (Mahieu, H. K. F. van Saene, et al., 1986, p. 324). As the organism is swallowed, it attaches mainly to the esophageal end of the prosthesis. Growths can start as early as 1 day after insertion of the prosthesis, and once the fungi have adhered to the silicone, it is almost impossible to remove them. Candida deterioration of the prosthesis can affect phonation by causing reduced loudness, unacceptable quality or pitch, shortened phonation time, aphonia, and increased resistance to airflow (Izdebski et al., 1987).

A variety of treatments have been suggested for decontaminating the host and the prosthesis. Mahieu, H. K. F. van Saene, et al. (1986) proposed that "yeasts can be reduced or eliminated from the oropharyngeal cavity by means of an oropharyngeal decontamination with amphotericin B lozenges" (p. 325). Furthermore, they suggested (a) coating the prosthesis with polymethyl methacrylates to lower the affinity of the candida organisms, or (b) impregnating the prosthesis with antimycotic agents or disinfectants. Blom and Singer (1986) advised disinfecting the prosthesis with nystatin or hydrogen peroxide rather than eradicating the organism from the host. Patients are instructed to remove the prosthesis every 3 days and submerge it in disinfectant overnight. The prosthesis can be reinserted after thorough rinsing. Although many patients begin candida treatment using hydrogen peroxide because it is relatively inexpensive and not a prescription item, if they do not have success, they should consider changing to nystatin. Izdebski et al. (1987) mentioned that "oral gargling with nystatin and brief soaking of the voice prosthesis may prevent colonization" of the candida organism (p. 597). I have observed successful treatment for control of candida in patients who swish and swallow one teaspoon of nystatin four times a day for 5 days, and soak their prosthesis in one teaspoon of nystatin for 5 min every 3 days. After the first 5 days on this program, only the soaking is continued.

Forward Movement of the Prosthesis

The patient may notice the prosthesis extending forward of the fistula entrance. In other words, it does not appear to be the close fit it once was. Two causes are possible: (a) the prosthesis could be too long, or (b) the fistula is closing at the esophageal end and pushing the prosthesis anteriorly. The first thing to do is remove the prosthesis and try to insert a catheter compatible with the diameter of the prosthesis being worn. If the catheter goes in easily, there is obviously no problem with the fistula closing. If, however, there is some resistance, or if a smaller catheter has to be used to penetrate the back of the fistula, then one must determine the causes for the stenosis or the closing of the esophageal end of the fistula. Recall that the fistula is in a constant state of closure, and this closure begins at the esophageal end and moves toward the tracheal end. Because the prosthesis keeps the fistula open, if the prosthesis is too short, the esophageal end may stenose or close. Also, the patient may dislodge the prosthesis by inadvertently catching and pulling on the prosthesis or neck strap while wiping away discharge. Lund, Perry, and Cheesman (1987) advised that patients who use a tracheostoma valve have to be careful when removing the valve housing or changing a stoma cover. The neck strap of the prosthesis may have adhesive residue on it, and may become dislodged by adhering to the housing or stoma cover. Vigorous sneezing or coughing also may dislodge a prosthesis, so when possible, the patient should place a finger across the top of the stoma to prevent forward movement of the prosthesis. Finally, the prosthesis may not have been inserted all the way into the esophagus.

If the fistula is open and the prosthesis extends 3–4 mm or more forward of the entrance, the prosthesis is too long and the patient should be measured for a shorter size. The difference between the standard sizes of the Blom–Singer and Bivona removeable prostheses ranges from 3 to 4 mm. Extension into the trachea can be observed during resting and swallowing, or with a slight forward pull on the neck strap of the prosthesis. The patient is likely to require down-sizing to a shorter prosthesis at least once, if not two or more times after the initial fitting.

Enlargement of Tissue Around the Fistula

Lund et al. (1987) described the formation of granulations around the tracheal opening of the fistula in some of their patients. The granulations are associated with crusting and bleeding, and are attributed to changing prostheses too infrequently. Lund et al. recommended treatment with "silver nitrate cautery (as an out-patient procedure) or by cryoprobe and occasionally removal of the voice prosthesis and insertion of the catheter for 48 hours" (p. 166). These authors also observed "soft tissue growth," described as a

> trunk of tissue [which] grows into the lumen of the fistula or around the prosthesis, pouting out into both the trachea and oesophagus at either end of the fistula and rendering use of the voice prosthesis difficult owing to occlusion of air flow and increasing the incidence of leakage. (p. 166)

Histology indicates chronic inflammation and fibrosis with ulceration along the track. Lund et al. advocated surgical removal of the growths or closure of the fistula with repuncture at a later date.

I have also observed several patients who have had doughnut-shaped growths form around the entrance to the fistula. The growth can extend the length of the fistula, requiring the patient to change to a longer prosthesis. The growth was surgically removed from one patient because it had become so large it compromised his airway. The pathology report on the tissue specimen revealed erosions, ulceration, and inflammation. There are clinical indications that this tissue formation may be related to irritation from the air entry port in the prosthesis, and possibly other irritating factors such as poor prosthesis hygiene or use of a prosthesis that is too long for the fistula. Treatment procedures that have met with varying success include electrocauterization and use of Elase ointment. The Elase ointment is applied to the growth with a cotton-tipped applicator, once a day for a week or longer, as determined by the physician. Changing to a prosthesis that has no air entry port seems to have been most helpful in containing further enlargement of the tissue. With the exception of the one surgically managed patient, the growths in the remaining patients have either remained stable (some over as long as 6 years) or reduced in size. It is advisable to recognize early that the air entry port on a prosthesis is in part or totally within the lumen of the fistula, and to change to a prosthesis without an air entry port as soon as possible.

CLOSURE OF THE FISTULA

Spontaneous Closure

Spontaneous closure may take place when (a) the prosthesis is too short for the length of the fistula, (b) the prosthesis has not been inserted completely, (c) the fistula is misaligned, or (d) the fistula wall is weak or collapsed. The first two causes and solutions are self-explanatory.

A misalignment of the fistula exists when the entrance of the fistula is not aligned with the exit. On inserting the prosthesis or catheter, one may experience a wall or increased resistance before reaching the esophageal end. With additional effort, the prosthesis may pass through this tight spot and enter the esophagus. One of my patients has described the sensation of inserting his prosthesis as "passing through two walls." Insertion and withdrawal of the prosthesis can be more or less difficult, depending upon the degree of misalignment. In some cases, it may be necessary to allow the fistula to close and perform another TEF procedure. Misalignment does not appear to improve over time. Sometimes it is helpful if the patient stents the fistula overnight with a catheter that is larger in diameter than would be necessary normally. This procedure seems to set up the fistula to hold a reasonable lumen long enough to insert the prosthesis without excessive difficulty.

The idea of a weakness or collapse of the fistula wall is speculative as nothing in the literature corroborates such a finding. I derived the notion from my experience with a patient who had his TEF when he was 78 years old. He did well with self-care for 2½ years, at which time he complained of having difficulty inserting his prosthesis. He up-stented first with a 16 Fr. catheter, and when the trouble persisted, used an 18 Fr. catheter for 20 min prior to each insertion of the prosthesis. Six months later, at age 81, he complained of difficulty removing the prosthesis as well as inserting it. In a diagnostic session, I found that insertion of a catheter met with resistance the length of the fistula; it seemed as if the tracheoesophageal wall had lost some of its tonus, possibly incident to aging, and was collapsing into the fistula. Furthermore, when the catheter was withdrawn, it was completely dry, suggesting lack of moisture in the tissues around the fistula. The results of fiberoptic endoscopy were normal. There appeared to be no way to resolve the resistance of the tissues to prosthesis withdrawal short of using a prosthesis without a retention collar. Such a prosthesis would not be a wise choice for this patient, whose prosthesis length was only 2.2 cm. The condition persists. The suggestions that have aided the patient's prosthesis insertion have been to: (a) stent the fistula with a well-lubricated 16 Fr. catheter for 5 min prior to insertion; (b) withdraw the catheter; (c) immediately pull upward on the neck tissue just above the stoma to expose and hold taut the fistula entrance, and maintain this position during prosthesis insertion; (d) promptly insert the prosthesis that has been generously lubricated with a water-soluble jelly. The patient soon will be 83 years old, and he has been able to continue using his TEF by following these procedures.

Planned Closure

Rationale. There are many reasons for considering letting the fistula close. In addition to medical problems, such as persistent leaking, inflammation, fibrosis, or ulceration associated with the fistula, the patient may not like the sound of his or her voice. The TEF sound may be rejected on the basis of pitch, quality, or loudness that does not meet expectations, match sex, or compare favorably to the patient's esophageal or artificial larynx speech. When the fistulization is part of the primary procedure, and the patient does not have the opportunity to use other methods of communication, the patient may compare the TEF sound only to laryngeal sound, and be dissatisfied with the results.

The patient also may reject the TEF because of the necessity for finger occlusion of the stoma. Some patients may need to have both hands free. Perhaps their jobs require them to be able to speak while working with both hands. If their hands get dirty, covering the stoma—even over a stoma cover—becomes unsanitary or unsightly. Patients who are food handlers may not be able to combine stoma occlusion with requirements for good hygiene. Unfortunately, professionals cannot determine before the surgery whether the patient will be able to use a tracheostoma valve successfully. Many patients will not be able to do so, and finger occlusion is the only other alternative at present.

Other reasons for considering fistula closure are concerned with management of the fistula and prosthesis. Visual acuity and manual dexterity may not have been considered prior to the TEF surgery, or changes in these functions may have occurred due to medical problems or aging, leaving the patient unable to care for the prosthesis easily. The patient may have been dependent upon a significant other to clean and insert the prosthesis, and that person is no longer available. Furthermore, lack of success with TEF has been correlated with alcohol abuse (Schuller, Jarrow, Kelly, & Miglets, 1983), which is confirmed by my clinical experience.

Procedures. Several methods promote closure of the fistula. A TEF that has been created by a surgical procedure based on the Singer–Blom technique is always trying to close. When given the opportunity, the fistula will close beginning at the esophageal end and moving toward the tracheal end. One way to provide the TEF opportunity to close is to remove the prosthesis at bedtime, and having nothing to eat or drink. Swallowing is infrequent during sleep, so leaking should not be a problem. By the next morning, the esophageal end of the fistula may be closed enough to allow normal intake of food and liquid with aspiration. Closure of the fistula may also be achieved in gradual steps by removing the prosthesis and replacing it with a series of catheters, each one smaller in diameter than the preceding one. For example, if a 14 Fr. catheter is compatible with the prosthesis being used, a 12 Fr. catheter could be inserted on the first night, a 10 Fr. on the next night, and the patient probably would be able to go without a catheter on the third night, and expect the fistula to be closed at the esophageal end by the following morning.

To determine whether the fistula has closed, the patient should try to produce sound by occluding the stoma and shunting air through the open fistula. If no sound is produced, the patient should swallow a small sip of water and observe the fistula entrance for leaking. If no leaking occurs, a larger sip is taken, and the fistula again observed for leaking. No sound and the absence of leaking on swallowing liquids means the esophageal end of the fistula has closed.

If a small leak persists for several days, the patient may need to have electrocauterization to complete the process. This procedure, done by a surgeon, takes only a few minutes under a local anesthetic. Generally only one treatment is needed, but occasionally more are required. A surgical closure of the fistula may need to be undertaken when the fistula fails to close, and/or the lumen enlarges to a permanent diameter that allows leaking between the prosthesis and the wall of the fistula (Andrews, Mickel, Hanson, Monahan, & Ward, 1987; Annyas & Escajadillo, 1984; Singer et al., 1981).

EMERGENCY PROCEDURES

Emergency Cards

Every individual who has a TEF must be knowledgeable about emergency procedures because many emergency rooms and physicians are unfamiliar with this surgery, and may not understand how to be of assistance. In addition to the emergency card available to all laryngectomees from the American Cancer Society, the society now has a card providing emergency information for tracheoesophageal fistula users. This card requires the patient to provide information appropriate to his or her unique requirements. Space is provided for the telephone numbers of the patient's physician and speech pathologist, should additional information be needed. The TEF patient must carry both cards.

Preventing Aspiration of Prosthesis

Occasionally a prosthesis is dropped or inhaled into the trachea. If it is not coughed out, it may be necessary to take the patient to the operating room to remove it. To prevent this from becoming a traumatic event, use a large, flat button, or drill a small hole near the edge of a poker chip. Take a needle and some strong thread, and attach either the button or the poker chip to the outside strap (wing) of the prosthesis. There should be about 5–6 in. of thread between the button or poker chip and the strap. The button or poker chip can be taped to the side of the neck to keep it out of the way. A prosthesis that enters the airway can now be retrieved easily.

Reopening the Fistula

If the fistula begins to close, the object is to try to get something into the fistula to keep it open, or, if it has already closed, to open it by penetrating the newly closed tissue. Start with a catheter that is the same size as that used to stent the opening for the prosthesis being worn (e.g., a 14 for a 16 Fr. prosthesis). The orange Rob-Nel catheters are stiffer, and consequently more penetrating than the red rubber ones. Insert the catheter into the fistula as far as it will go. One can assume that the catheter is in the esophagus if it passes easily and without discomfort to within 4 or 5 in. of the outside end. If it does not enter the esophagus, apply *continuous and mildly forceful pressure for several minutes.* If the catheter does not penetrate through to the esophagus, try the next smaller size catheter, using the same procedure. It may be necessary to use a 10 Fr. or smaller to penetrate the closure.

Opening a closed fistula can take some time, so patience is necessary. The newly closed tissue should give way first and keep the catheter from creating a new fistula; unfortunately, sometimes a new fistula is created. The patient will know when the catheter is not following the path of the old fistula because there will be pain which may become severe if the probing continues. Another sign is when the catheter has been inserted 1½ in. or more and is still not in the esophagus. *There should be no significant pain or discomfort on probing with the catheter, and little or no bleeding.* The patient should be aware only of the pressure being exerted against the tissues.

If the catheter does enter the esophagus, a knot should be tied about 4 in. from the outside end to prevent leakage. Tape the catheter to the side of the neck. The patient should contact his or her physician or speech pathologist for further advice as soon as possible. The fistula can be up-stented with sequentially larger catheters until the catheter size is compatible with the size of the prosthesis. It may take 3 hr or so between catheters, or each catheter may have to be in overnight. It is sometimes possible to up-stent faster by skipping a size.

If the catheter can be inserted only part of the way, the fistula may still be salvageable if the catheter is kept inserted as far as it will go, and the patient proceeds immediately to the physician, speech pathologist, or emergency room, taking all the personal supplies used for the tracheoesophageal fistula, including prostheses, catheters, tape and other adhesives, and inserters. The physician may wish to try other procedures.

Patient Kit

The patient should have catheters ranging in size from about 10 Fr., which is small, to the largest size used when the prosthesis is inserted. Sets of these catheters should be kept at home, in the car, at the office, and so forth, to be used for any emergency. The patient should be able to keep the fistula open regardless of any problem with the prosthesis. Additional supplies to consider for an emergency kit include a spare prosthesis, adhesive tape, scissors, pipe cleaners, cotton-tipped applicators, and possibly some liquid silicone adhesive.

AUTHOR'S COMMENT

The information in this chapter is based largely on personal experience with patients, using the technology available up to the time of this writing. However, the new field of tracheoesophageal fistulization continues to grow and change as it attracts worldwide attention and research. Practical information will most assuredly be affected. Therefore, concerned professionals must be attuned to new developments, remain flexible in their approach, and examine new surgeries, prostheses, and therapeutic procedures critically and without bias.

REFERENCES

Andrews, J. C., Mickel, R. A., Hanson, D. G., Monahan, G. P., & Ward, P. H. (1987). Major complications following tracheoesophageal puncture for voice rehabilitation. *Laryngoscope, 97,* 562–567.

Annyas, A. A., & Escajadillo, J. R. (1984). Closure of tracheoesophageal fistulas after removal of the voice prosthesis. *Laryngoscope, 94,* 1244–1245.

Blom, E. D. (1989). *Voice restoration after laryngectomy.* Paper presented at VA Medical Center Seminar, Martinsburg, WV.

Blom, E. D., & Singer, M. I. (1986). Disinfection of silicone voice prostheses. *Archives of Otolaryngology–Head and Neck Surgery, 112,* 1303.

Izdebski, K., Ross, J. C., & Lee, S. (1987). Fungal colonization of tracheoesophageal voice prosthesis. *Laryngoscope, 97,* 594–597.

Lund, V. J., Perry, A., & Cheesman, A. D. (1987). Blom–Singer puncture (practicalities in everyday management). *Journal of Laryngology and Otology, 101,* 164–168.

Mahieu, H. F., Rosingh, H. J., Saene, R. K., & Schutte, H. K. (1985). Deterioration of voice prostheses caused by fungal vegetations [Letter to the editor]. *Archives of Otolaryngology, 111,* 280.

Mahieu, H. F., van Saene, H. K. F., Rosingh, H. J., & Schutte, H. K. (1986). Candida vegetations on silicone voice prostheses. *Archives of Otolaryngology–Head and Neck Surgery, 112,* 321–325.

Mahieu, H. F., van Saene, J. J. M., den Besten, J., & van Saene, H. K. F. (1986). Oropharynx decontamination preventing Candida vegetation on voice prostheses. *Archives of Otolaryngology–Head and Neck Surgery, 112,* 1090–1092.

Modica, L. A. (1987). Care of tracheoesophageal voice prostheses [Letter to the editor]. *Archives of Otolaryngology–Head and Neck Surgery, 113,* 436.

Rodu, B., Griffin, I. L., & Gockerman, J. P. (1984). Oral candidiasis in cancer patients. *Southern Medical Journal, 77,* 312–314.

Schuller, D. E., Jarrow, J. E., Kelly, D. R., & Miglets, A. W. (1983). Prognostic factors affecting the success of duckbill voice restoration. *Otolaryngology and Head and Neck Surgery, 91,* 396–398.

Shagets, F. W., & Panje, W. R. (1985). Primary tracheoesophageal fistula formation for feeding and voice rehabilitation. *Laryngoscope, 95,* 1001–1003.

Singer, M. I., & Blom, E. D. (1980). An endoscopic technique for restoration of voice after laryngectomy. *Annals of Otology, Rhinology and Laryngology, 89,* 529–533.

Singer, M. I., Blom, E. D., & Hamaker, R. C. (1981). Further experience with voice restoration after total laryngectomy. *Annals of Otology, Rhinology and Laryngology, 90,* 498–502.

Smith, B. E. (1986). Aerodynamic characteristics of Blom–Singer low pressure voice prostheses. *Archives of Otolaryngology–Head and Neck Surgery, 112,* 50–52.

Weinberg, B., & Moon, J. (1984). Aerodynamic properties of four tracheoesophageal puncture prostheses. *Archives of Otolaryngology, 110,* 673–675.

Weinberg, B., & Moon, J. (1986a). Airway resistances of Blom–Singer and Panje low pressure tracheoesophageal puncture prostheses. *Journal of Speech and Hearing Disorders, 51,* 169–172.

Weinberg, B., & Moon, J. (1986b). Impact of tracheoesophageal puncture prosthesis airway resistance on in-vivo phonatory performance. *Journal of Speech and Hearing Disorders, 51,* 88–91.

CHAPTER 8

Clinical Application of Alaryngeal Speech Judgments

Mary A. Carpenter

Carpenter presents an extensive review of studies concerned with perceptual judgments of proficiency/preference in alaryngeal speech. She discusses the role of perceptual judgments in speech training and their relative importance in influencing treatment decisions. Carpenter cautions clinicians that the usefulness of the data is limited. Clinicians will be challenged by alternative guidelines she proposes for organizing and terminating treatment.

Study Questions

1. What variables should be considered in evaluating alaryngeal speech proficiency/preference to assure representativeness of the data?
2. Which subskills affecting proficiency/preference are common across all alaryngeal speech types?
3. Why are proficiency judgments insufficient as a measure of success in alaryngeal speech training?

As in any treatment program, ongoing evaluation is critical in alaryngeal speech rehabilitation. Measures of individual skills obviously are part of treatment assessment; however, at some point, it must be determined whether these isolated skills combine to provide the desired outcome. This evaluation is particularly relevant in alaryngeal speech training because of the unique need to restructure an entire communication process. Perceptual measures have been preferred for this composite index, given their ability to reflect overall speech performance and to represent the speaker–listener interaction.

Although various labels have been used to describe these perceptual measures, they reduce to two primary categories, *judgments of preference* and *judgments of proficiency,* each reflecting a somewhat different focus. Preference judgments reflect the *listener's reaction* (dependent variable) to the speech performance; proficiency judgments describe the *speaker's performance* (the dependent variable where the listener is merely the measurement vehicle). For both, data typically are acquired through scaled scores or through some form of relative comparison. Although these measures of preference and proficiency would seem to be positively correlated, each reflects a separate part of the communication dyad: the speaker or the listener.

Another perceptual measure, *intelligibility,* also is used as a broad performance index. Although potentially viewed as a component of speaker proficiency, intelligibility clearly depends on the perception of the listener. As such, it presents a combination of the two primary judgment categories and has proved a popular alternative. Data typically are reported as percentages and can reflect everything from phoneme to concept recognition.

The purpose of this chapter is not to describe how to generate these composite perceptual measures of preference, proficiency, and intelligibility, but rather to discuss their application in alaryngeal speech training. To provide a framework, the material is divided into sections based on the primary questions addressed in treatment planning. Each unit begins with a brief overview of the applicable decision process, with the role of these perceptual measures identified. Then, because decisions can be influenced both by data unique to the client and by observations universal to the population, the related research is summarized in tabular form and briefly in text. Closing comments address clinical application, with special attention given to problems in utilization of the literature. For convenience, the abbreviations TE, ES, and AL are used throughout this chapter to represent *tracheoesophageal, esophageal,* and *artificial larynx,* respectively.

As a precursor to what follows, a few comments are in order. First, the models/guidelines offered for treatment represent only one alternative for structuring the decision processes. Other forms exist; however, the role of overall performance measures remains roughly the same in each. Second, no pretense is made concerning completeness of the research reviews and critiques. Some selectivity was intentional; some may reflect oversight. Liberties also were taken in extrapolating, categorizing, and interpreting the data to suit the focus of this chapter. Apologies are due referenced authors if this attempt at organization led to misrepresentation.

TYPE OF SPEECH

Decision Guidelines

Determining the form of alaryngeal communication to be used is the most fundamental and pervasive of the decisions structuring treatment. Alternatives are compared on the basis of the individual's speech potential, the anticipated speech setting, and the eventual acquired speech product (see Figure 8.1). Certain factors will have similar influence regardless of speech type; others may affect only particular alternatives. Relative evaluation of these components establishes not only the appropriateness of oral versus nonoral communication, but also the suitability of the major speech options (TE, ES, AL) and/or alternatives within types (e.g., different ALs).

Review of the client's *speech potential* begins at the preoperative contact and continues into the initial postoperative instruction. Beyond

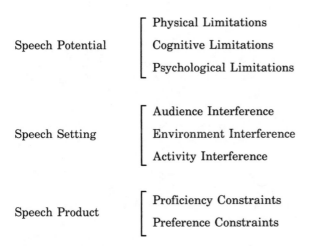

Figure 8.1. Factors considered in selection of alaryngeal communication alternatives.

basic consideration of availability of services and supplies, emphasis is on the client's physical, cognitive, and psychological limitations. Factors are considered with respect to demands of the particular speech type and the training involved.

In considering *speech setting,* the focus is on sources of interference in the audience (e.g., hearing loss), the environment (e.g., noise), and the activity involved (e.g., hands required). Relevant factors can be anticipated to some extent, although some will become apparent only over time. Since contexts are likely to vary, priority is given to those that occur with greatest frequency or carry most importance.

Evaluation of the *speech product* addresses constraints both in the overt performance (proficiency) and in the reactions to performance (preference). Outcomes may be predetermined in some respects; however, because a priori estimates may be inaccurate or incomplete, assessment occurs after minimal skills are established and continues for the duration of the program. Initial emphasis is on proficiency since it appears to be a legitimate prerequisite to preference.

The intent of this evaluation is not to isolate a single speech alternative. More appropriately, the purpose is to rule out options that are not feasible and to define relative merits of the remaining speech types. Obviously, composite perceptual measures are utilized in this decision sequence to evaluate the speech product. Proficiency and preference data are generated for the client using each speech type and are compared to identify relative strengths; however, consideration of the related research also could influence this selection process if the evidence clearly favors certain alternatives.

Literature Review

Research addressing the relative merits of the various forms of alaryngeal speech has been based on both measures of intelligibility and measures of preference. In most cases, comparison has been made across the primary speech types of AL, TE, and ES, although a few studies consider contrasts within type (e.g., different forms of ALs). Methodologies differ markedly among studies, with one critical distinction being that some studies used different speakers for each speech option whereas others replicated speakers across speech types.

The following review is organized according to these divisions based on the type of measure applied and the design used. Selected articles were limited to those that directly contrast speech alternatives, since comparison of studies of single speech types invites risks in interpretation. Findings are summarized across studies without strict limitation to statistically significant outcomes. This approach was adopted both because of the emphasis on common patterns and because of the absence of such analysis in some cases.

Intelligibility.   *Between type.*   At face value, within-subject studies of relative intelligibility between speech types reflect a mixed performance in comparing ES and AL speakers, but a consistently superior performance for TE over AL speakers. Within-subject comparisons of ES and TE speech reflect equal or greater intelligibility for the latter. (See Table 8.1.)

Between-subject studies indicate that where differences exist, the intelligibility of TE speech typically is equal or superior to both AL and ES alternatives. (See Table 8.2.) When judgments are made in noise, or are provided by older listeners, AL speech predominates. This influence of listening condition and listener type is limited, however, to studies of single speakers for each speech option. Between-subject comparisons of only AL and ES speech suggest equal or greater intelligibility for the latter, with some influence from the listener group on the outcome.

Within type.   Intelligibility studies within speech type all are based on within-subject comparisons of AL speech across commercial alternatives (see Table 8.3). Little value is gained in attempting to summarize across studies by instrument since most considered different ALs, and in different manners. If the data are reviewed simply to identify whether differences occurred among instruments regardless of type, then mixed patterns appear. There is some indication, however, that the differences reported in intelligibility are dependent on variables other than the instrument involved (e.g., the stimulus or the form of measurement).

Preference.   *Between type.*   Within-subject studies of listener preference across speech type are few in number and have considered restricted alternatives and speaker populations (see Table 8.4). However, findings appear grossly similar to those for between-subject studies, where TE speech reportedly is equal or superior to AL and ES based on listener perception (see Table 8.5). No common pattern exists for the comparisons of ES and AL speech, although there is some suggestion that the preference status of the latter is contingent on the particular instrument used.

Within type.   Investigations of listener preference within speech type typically are restricted to within-subject studies of various ALs (see Table 8.6). Again, since the studies are dissimilar with respect to the devices used and are limited in the number of speakers studied, conclusions regarding specific AL preferences are discouraged. There is strong indication, however, that different devices do provoke differences in preference. It also is interesting to note that discrepancies in preference may occur between listeners and speakers, and among speakers, for the same sample.

TABLE 8.1
Intelligibility Comparisons Between Alaryngeal Speech Types (Within Subjects)

	Speakers	Measure	Medium	Listeners	Results AL	Results ES	Results TE
Golper & Rau (1978)	6 AL (6) ES	Sentence Transcription	AV	12 Students (Speech Pathology)	1 2 =	2 1 =	(N=3) (N=2) (N=1)
Kalb & Carpenter (1981)	5 AL[a] (5) ES	Word Transcription	A	30 Students (Naive)	=	=	
Wetmore et al. (1981)	11 AL (11) TE	Scaled (sample?)	?	?	2		1
Goldstein et al. (1984)	7 AL 1 ES (8) TE	Word Choice	A	45 Students	2		1
Blom et al. (1986)	27 AL (27) TE	Word Choice	AV	80 Naive (5/speaker)	2		1
	7 ES (7) TE	Word Choice	AV	80 Naive (5/speaker)		=	=
Doyle et al. (1988)	1 ES (1) TE	Word Transcription	A	15 Naive		2	1
	1 ES (1) TE	Scaled Monologue	A	15 Naive		=	=

Note. AL = artificial larynx. ES = esophageal. TE = tracheoesophageal. AV = audiovisual. A = audio. Results are shown in rank order where 1 = Best. [a]Described as using same AL type.

TABLE 8.2
Intelligibility Comparisons Between Alaryngeal Speech Types (Between Subjects)

	Speakers	Measure	Medium	Listeners	Results		
					AL	ES	TE
Williams & Watson (1984)	11 AL	Scaled (varied sample)	AV	3 Naive	3	2	1
	12 ES			3 Informed	3	2	1
	10 TE			3 Expert	=	=	1
Clark (1985)	1 AL	Synthetic Sentence Choice	A:0dB S:N	11 Young	=	=	=
	1 ES			11 Old	1	=	=
	1 TE		−5dB S:N	11 Young	1	2	3
				11 Old	1	=	=
			−10dB S:N	11 Young	1	2	3
				11 Old	1	2	3
Hyman (1955)	8 AL[a]	Word Choice	A	120 Students	=	=	
	8 ES	Syllable Transcription	A	7 Students	=	=	

Table continues

TABLE 8.2 Continued

	Speakers		Measure	Medium	Listeners	Results		
						AL	ES	TE
McCroskey & Mulligan (1963)	5	AL	Word	A	10 Naive	=	=	
	5	ES	Choice		10 Exposed	2	1	
					10 Expert	2	1	
Shames et al. (1963)	35	AL	Word	A	5 Students	2	1	
	19	ES	Transcription					
	12	AL	Key Word	A	5 Students	=	=	
	31	ES	Transcription					
Kalb & Carpenter (1981)	5	AL[a]	Word	A	30 Students	2	1	
	5	ES	Transcription					
Doyle et al. (1988)	3	ES	Word	A	15 Naive		2	1
	3	TE	Transcription					
			Scaled	A	15 Naive		2	1
			Monologue					

Note. AL = artificial larynx. ES = esophageal. TE = tracheoesophageal. AV = audiovisual. A = audio. Results are shown in rank order where 1 = Best. [a]Described as using same AL type.

TABLE 8.3

Intelligibility Comparisons Within Alaryngeal Speech Types (All Within Subject; All Artificial Larynx)

Speakers	Listeners	Medium	Measure	Diff.	No Diff.
Zwitman & Disinger (1975) 1 C-R oral (1) WE oral	4 ?	AV?	Transcriptions:		
			Sents. (Type A)	X	
			Words (Type A)		X
			Sents. (Type B)		X
Goshorn & Schinsky (1976) 9 WE neck (9) WE oral (9) C-R oral	9 Experienced (1/Speaker)	A?	Rank Order	X	but
			Word Choice	X	different outcomes
Zwitman et al. (1978) 2 Intraoral (2) Transoral	7 ?	AV	Word Transcrip.		X
			Sent. Transcrip.		X
Stalker et al. (1982) 1 WE 5A (1) WE 5B (1) Aurex (1) Servox (1) Barts	28 Naive	AV	Word Choice	X	
			Key Word Transcription		X
Weiss & Basili (1985) 6 WE 5 (6) Servox	6 Experienced	A	Word Transcription		X
Anderson (1986) 3 WE 5-I (3) WE 5-II (3) WE 5-III	30 Naive	A	Word Transcription		X

Note. C-R = Cooper-Rand. WE = Western Electric. AV = audiovisual. A = audio. Results are shown only as Difference/No Difference among AL types.

TABLE 8.4
Preference Comparisons Between Alaryngeal Speech Types (Within Subject)

Speakers	Measure	Medium	Listeners	Results AL	ES	TE
Green & Hults (1982)						
1 AL (x) (1) AL (y) (1) ES	Scaled (counting, spontaneous)	AV	75 Naive	1(x) 2(y)	3	
			38 Sp. Path	1(x) 3(y)	2	
Goldstein et al. (1984)						
7 AL 1 ES (8) TE	Paired Comparison (sentences)	A	45 Students	2		1
Blom et al. (1986)						
27 AL (27) TE	Scaled (paragraph)	AV	80 Naive (5/speaker)	2		1
7 ES (7) TE	Scaled (paragraph)	AV	80 Naive (5/speaker)		2	1

Note. AL = artificial larynx. ES = esophageal. TE = tracheoesophageal. AV = audiovisual. A = audio. (x) and (y) represent different artificial larynges. Results are shown in rank order where 1 = Most Preferred.

TABLE 8.5

Preference Comparisons Between Alaryngeal Speech Types (Between Subjects)

	Samples	Measure	Medium	Listeners	Results AL	Results ES	Results TE
Clark & Stemple (1982)	1 AL 1 ES 1 TE	Rank Order (sentence)	A	20 ?	[2]	[3]	[1]
Hyman (1955)	8 AL[a] 8 ES	Paired-Comparison (sentence)	A	100 Students	1	2	
Crouse (1962; cited in Goldstein, 1978)	5 AL 5 ES	? (passage)	AV A	12 Professional 12 Naive	2 2	1 1	
Bennett & Weinberg (1973)	1 AL (x) 2 AL (y) 2 AL (z) 5 ES	Scaled (sentence)	A	37 Naive	1(x) 3(y,z)	2	
Trudeau (1987)	13 ES 12 TE	Scaled (sentences)	A	25 Naive		=	=

Note. AL = artificial larynx. ES = esophageal. TE = tracheoesophageal. AV = audiovisual. A = audio. (x), (y), and (z) represent different artificial larynges. Results are shown in rank order where 1 = Most Preferred. [a]Described as using same AL type. [ ] = not significant.

TABLE 8.6
Preference Comparisons Within Alaryngeal Speech Types (Between/Within Subjects)

	Samples	Measure	Medium	Listeners	Results Diff.	Results No Diff.
Bennett & Weinberg (1973)	AL: 1 Bell 5A 2 WE Reed 1 Tokyo	Scaled (sentence)	A	37 Naive	X	
Green & Hults (1982)	AL: 1 Tokyo (1) Servox	Scaled (count & spontaneous)	AV	75 Naive 38 Sp. Path.	X X	
Stalker et al. (1982)	AL: 1 WE 5A (1) WE 5B (1) Aurex (1) Servox (1) Barts	Scaled (paragraph)	AV	28 Naive	X	
Anderson (1986)	AL: 3 WE 5-I (3) WE 5-II (3) WE 5-III	Rank Order (sentences)	Live	3 Speakers	X	(diff. choice per speaker)
Henley-Cohn et al. (1984)	TE: 8 Bivona (8) Panje (8) Henley-Cohn et al.	Rank Order (?)	Live	8 Speakers	X	(same choice for spkrs.)
Blom et al. (1986)	TE: 20 No TSV 24 With TSV	Scaled (paragraph)	AV	80 Naive (5/speaker)	X	

Note. AL = artificial larynx. TE = tracheoesophageal. WE = Western Electric. TSV = tracheostomal valve. A = audio. AV = audiovisual. Results are shown only as Difference/No Difference among AL/TE types. ( ) = within subject.

Clinical Application

At face value, this literature might be interpreted as favoring use of TE over AL or ES speech (except under select conditions) if consideration is given solely to the speech product. If the choice is between AL and ES speech, dominance of speech type is less clear. Indications are that the outcome may differ depending on the speaker, the type of stimuli used in the evaluation, and the listening audience. The literature also does not identify a particular AL of choice by type. The findings do suggest, however, that differences between instruments should be expected, but, again, not consistently across speech stimuli or listener groups.

Application of this information in selection of speech type is appropriate only to the degree that these studies are representative of the clinical decision. Particularly critical to clinical application is the questionable assumption that between-subject differences will parallel the within-subject comparisons made for a particular client. Although within-subject studies exist, they are limited in quantity, number of subjects studied, and variety of alternatives compared. Consideration also needs to be given to the similarity between the populations studied and the intended clinical case. In the majority of the articles reviewed, speakers and listeners are representative of only a particular subtype (e.g., "superior" speakers, "naive" listeners). If the client and expected audience do not parallel these populations, generalization of findings is suspect.

Other issues in representativeness also raise questions about the applicability of this research to clinical decisions. Specifically, concerns exist in generalizing from these studies since many are based on limited numbers of speakers and/or listeners, limited evidence of speaker reliability, and limited breadth of the speech samples. Even the representativeness of a single sample of each AL type is questionable, given the possible influence of adjustments in frequency, intensity, and tone settings.

In addition to these qualifiers is the issue of potential influence from procedural variables. Questions exist as to the impact of sample type, listener type, listening condition (the medium), and listener's task. Since these factors may have affected the studies' outcomes, interpretation is restricted to the conditions used. (Although not within the scope of this chapter, articles are available that describe the measured effects of many of these variables.)

Admittedly, these constraints in the literature do not call into question the validity of the research that has been done; however, they do affect clinical applicability. Regardless, the fundamental question may be moot since one could argue that there is little reason to expect major

174 Mary A. Carpenter174 Mary A. Carpenter

differences in proficiency among alaryngeal speech types for an individ-ual client. If the prerequisites have been carefully considered and themechanics well established, the remaining variables would seem to bethe noisy voice/sound source, which is inherent to all speech types, andthe articulatory patterns of the speaker, which would be similar acrosstypes. Differences in preference could emerge, however, given the con-trasts in auditory/visual naturalness between the speech alternatives.

For any one client, then, selection of speech type appears to be heav-ily dependent on demonstration of the prerequisites and the individual'spersonal preference. These two factors alone can narrow the options toa single alternative. Even if more than one speech type remains avail-able, rarely are all three primary alternatives represented. Optionsusually reduce to AL and TE *or* ES speech, but not both. Given thespeech types' different assets and liabilities, a case typically is madefor combined use of AL and TE or ES speech, either at different timesin the recovery process or in different settings.

Consequently, comparative evaluations of speech types may havelimited clinical utility, although they are applicable in some cases toestablish relative strengths between primary speech types or amongAL/prosthetic alternatives. For these cases, and even for assessment ofsingle speech alternatives over time, the literature does indirectly accentcertain procedural guidelines for perceptual evaluations of proficiency

1. Use speech samples representative of the client's performance, forexample, having adequate length and breadth.
2. Select samples representative of the expected speech needs, forinstance, with characteristic content and style.
3. Choose listeners representative of the predicted audience, with com-parable familiarity and visual/auditory acuity.
4. Test under conditions representative of the anticipated environment,for example, with similar noise levels and visibility.

Specifying a set of conditions applicable to all clients is difficult sincecritical factors will vary for each individual. The clinician is encouragedto test under the most varied conditions possible, however, to assureadequate representation. In most cases, it is appropriate to test bothwith and without visual cues, using samples with both high and lowlinguistic predictability, and including both familiar and unfamiliarlisteners or evaluators. Regardless of the conditions selected for eachclient, the clinician is strongly advised to replicate the measures for aparticular speech type and to duplicate conditions when testing acrossspeech types. Although representative conditions cannot always be anticipated for the individual, the validity of the data that are generated should be assured.

SUBSKILLS REQUIRED

Decision Guidelines

After deciding which speech modes are to be trained, identifying the relevant subskills is the next major decision in speech retraining. Since alaryngeal speech represents substitution of a totally new communication process, multiple factors must be considered. However, knowing which speech parameters are most critical to the final product not only increases treatment efficiency, but maximizes treatment effectiveness.

Broadly defined, the categories of subskills required for the final speech product are identical across speech types (see Figure 8.2), as would be expected given their common end goal. In each case, establishing the mechanics for consistent sound/voice production is the necessary first step. Obviously, the particular components to be considered depend on the type of speech being applied. Once the mechanics are mastered, attention is directed to controlling characteristics of the sound produced, including timing and duration.

The next two major categories focus not on sound/voice generation, but on parameters of speech. Arbitrary division is made here between features affecting intelligibility and those affecting naturalness. Although the distinction is useful, it is suspect since certain subskills such as rate, phrasing, and intonation can influence both categories. Subskills within these categories are essentially identical across speech types, but mechanisms for manipulation may differ.

The last category, loosely labeled speech distractions, also remains common to all speech types if broadly defined. Again, because of the unique processes involved, potential problems are typically specific to a speech type; however, features associated with excessive effort have some universality.

Given the multiple components involved in reestablishing speech, the consideration of subskills often appears overwhelming. However, direct training may not be required. In some cases skills emerge spontaneously, develop after minimal rehearsal, or result as a function of training in other areas. In addition, certain subskills may not be modifiable, at least not without negatively affecting other aspects of speech.

Some components can have limited impact on the overall product, which argues for reduced attention in treatment. Composite performance measures may be of assistance in this task of determining which sub-

	Artificial Larynx	Esophageal	Tracheoesophageal
Production of Sound	Placement/Seal Activation	Air Intake Air Return	Respiratory Drive Stoma Seal/Pressure
Control of Sound	Timing Loudness Quality Pitch	Duration Loudness Quality Pitch	Duration Loudness Quality Pitch
Intelligibility of Speech	Oral Pressure Voicing Contrasts Rate	Oral Pressure Voicing Contrasts Rate	Oral Pressure Voicing Contrasts Rate
Naturalness of Speech	Phrasing Pause Stress Intonation	Phrasing Pause Stress Intonation	Phrasing Pause Stress Intonation
Distractions to Speech	Stoma Noise Arm Posture (Etc.)	Stoma Noise Intake Noise (Etc.)	Stoma Leak Hand Posture (Etc.)

Figure 8.2. Production components for alaryngeal speech alternatives.

skills should have less or more weight. If a particular voice/speech feature can be systematically manipulated, its effect on judgments of proficiency and/or preference can be determined and the need for modification established. Of potential value, too, would be research evaluating the contribution of these factors to composite perceptual judgments.

Literature Review

As with the studies comparing speech types, some studies attempting to identify critical features in alaryngeal speech address correlates of proficiency, whereas others use acceptability or some other index of preference. Factors vary but they can be categorized loosely into those associated with voice and those associated with speech, with separate attention to phonemic error patterns. In all but one case, the studies are exclusive to a particular alaryngeal speech type.

The review also is organized according to speech type, although alternatives are combined within the tables to allow comparison. The distinction between proficiency and preference is temporarily ignored, however, given the limited volume of literature utilizing each measure and their presumed relationship. Studies typically are restricted to those that compare across speakers of different performance levels, since descriptions based solely on superior speakers may simply reflect the population at large. To further minimize error in interpretation, this review also focuses on research that utilizes direct measures of sample contrasts rather than listener impressions of distinguishing features. As before, and with similar rationale, findings are presented as a composite across studies without strict regard for statistical significance.

Esophageal Speech. *Voice.* Investigations of vocal features associated with levels of esophageal speech skill address fundamental frequency, intensity, quality, and degree of extraneous noise (see Table 8.7). Unfortunately, extrapolation is questionable given the limited data, limited similarity in features studied, and, in some cases, contradictory findings. Only one feature—fundamental frequency—was considered by all studies in this category. Results are mixed, although the majority reflect a positive relationship between frequency level and perceived skill. The only other replicated result indicates a lack of relationship between frequency variation and composite speech performance; however, the inconsistencies between these studies with regard to findings for other voice parameters make even this parallel suspect.

Speech. Characteristics of ES speech considered in relation to preference/proficiency encompass a variety of factors clustering in categories of duration, rate, pause, and intelligibility/articulation (see Table 8.8). Findings are relatively consistent and indicate a positive association between judged performance level and both duration of response per intake and rate of speech. Positive relationships also are typically identified with intelligibility/articulation. Pause time, whether measured as number of interruptions or proportion of total time, is negatively correlated.

Phonemes. Unfortunately, no studies are available comparing phoneme error patterns for differing ES proficiency levels. However, data can be considered across studies under the assumption that evidence of repeated patterns might indicate commonalities regardless of skill level (see Table 8.9). Comparisons are difficult because of the dissimilarities in forms of phonemic analysis and the different error patterns described. Regardless, common elements suggest more error on consonants than on vowels and for voiceless than for voiced phonemes. Frequency of error also appears to vary relative to manner of production, with greater error typically on fricatives and plosives than on affricates and glides. Some studies, however, indicate no differences relative to voicing and manner. Syllable position influence is equivocal.

TABLE 8.7

Voice Parameters Associated with Composite Esophageal and Artificial Larynx Speech Judgments

Esophageal	Sample N	Composite Judgment	Frequency Mean	Frequency Variance	Intensity/SPL Mean	Intensity/SPL Variance	Periodicity/ Consistency	Respiratory Noise/Klunk
Shipp (1967)	33	Acceptability	+	0			+	−
Hoops & Noll (1969)	22	Effectiveness	0	0	0	0	0	
Filter & Hyman (1975)	20	Effectiveness	+		+			

Artificial Larynx	Sample N	Composite Judgment	Frequency Mean	Frequency Variance	Intensity/SPL Mean	Intensity/SPL Variance	Noise/S:N
Weiss et al. (1979)	5 (normal)	(Preferred Speech Quality)			0		0
Kelly (1979)	1 (model)	Preference	−			0	
Rothman (1978)	15	Proficiency		0		+	−

Note. + = Positive association. − = Negative association. 0 = No association.

TABLE 8.8
Speech Parameters Associated with Composite Esophageal and Artificial Larynx Speech Judgments

Esophageal	Sample N	Composite Judgment	Syllable/Intake Units/Phrase	Rate	Pause (Amount)	Intelligibility	Articulation
Shipp (1967)	33	Acceptability		+	−		
Berlin (1965)	62	Acceptability	+				
Hoops & Noll (1969)	22	Effectiveness		+			
Filter & Hyman (1975)	20	Effectiveness		+		+	+
Berlin (1963)	38	Proficiency	+				
Creech (1966)	48	Proficiency				+	
Hoops & Guzek (1974)	40	Proficiency	+	+			

Artificial Larynx	Sample N	Composite Judgment		Rate	Pause (Location)	Intelligibility	
Weiss et al. (1979)	5 (normal)	(Preferred Speech Quality)		0		0	
Rothman (1978)	15	Proficiency		+	−		

Note. + = Positive association. − = Negative association. 0 = No association.

TABLE 8.9

Phoneme Error Patterns for Esophageal, Artificial Larynx, and Tracheoesophageal Speech Based on Type (Consonant/Vowel), Position (Initial/Final), Voicing (Voiceless/Voiced), and Manner

	Speaker N	Type C vs. V	Position I vs. F	Voicing Vl vs. Vd	Manner Most → Least
Esophageal					
Hyman (1955)	8	C	F	Vl	f p n g a
Sacco et al. (1967)	19	C		Vl	f p p n =
Horii & Weinberg (1975)	2	C	=	=	=
Doyle et al. (1988)	3			= (all stim.) Vl (cognates)	f =n =p a g
Artificial Larynx					
Hyman (1955)	8	C	F		p g f n a
Weiss et al. (1979)	5	C	I (f,p,a,g) F (n)	Vl (p:I) = (f,n,a,g)	p f a n g (I) f n p a g (F)
Cady (1981)	7 Hi; 7 Lo Intellig.		= (Hi Group) F (Lo Group)	Vl	f p a n g
Weiss & Basili (1985)	12	C	I (n,g) F (f,p,a)	Vl	f p a n g (I) f n p a g (F)

Table continues

TABLE 8.9 Continued

Speaker N	Type C vs. V	Position I vs. F	Voicing Vl vs. Vd	Manner Most ———— Least
Tracheoesophageal				
Doyle & Haaf (1987) 5		I (f,p,a) = (n,g)	Vl (p:l) = (f)	p f a n g (I) f a n p g (F)
Doyle et al. (1988) 3			Vl	a f p n g

Note. Areas of greater error are indicated or shown in rank order. f = fricative, p = plosive, a = affricate, n = nasal, g = glide.

Artificial Larynx Speech. *Voice.* Voice parameters considered in AL speech are similar to those addressed in ES performance (see Table 8.7). Unfortunately, constraints to extrapolation also are similar. In this case, no findings were replicated across studies, precluding identification of patterns.

Speech. Components of AL speech selected for study somewhat parallel those considered for ES speech (see Table 8.8). However, the limited volume of research and the discrepant findings are more like those reported for features of voice. Constraints again are sufficient to preclude interpretation, although it is tempting to predict that findings would be similar to those for ES speech with a larger data base.

Phonemes. In the case of AL articulation, one study does contrast performances of two speaker groups of different intelligibility levels (Cady, 1981) (see Table 8.9). In general, frequency and error type were highly similar for the two groups, strengthening the argument for comparing across studies as was done with the ES data. As before, collated descriptions are difficult to derive, but some patterns do emerge. Again, more errors occur on consonants than on vowels and, typically, for voiceless than for voiced phonemes. Evidence relative to consonant position in a syllable is mixed, with some indication that it may be influenced by manner of production. Description of error patterns relative to manner are reasonably consistent with greater error reported for fricatives/plosives than for nasals/glides. This rank order diverges somewhat between studies, possibly reflecting the interaction between manner and syllable position noted earlier. However, differences in manner classifications even within studies tend to be small, except possibly between the extremes.

Tracheoesophageal Speech. Insufficient data are available to identify voice/speech characteristics associated with various skill levels in TE speakers. However, because of the similarity to ES and AL speech patterns, a description of TE phonemic errors is included, although findings are limited to two studies (see Table 8.9).

In TE speech, as in other alaryngeal speech types, phonemic error patterns emerge relative to consonant position, voicing, and manner of production. In this case, errors are more pronounced in prevocalic than postvocalic contexts, and more frequent on voiceless than voiced phonemes. With respect to manner of production, errors tend to occur most often on fricatives/affricates and least often on nasals/glides, with some variation in the rank order of plosives. As noted, however, the data base for this extrapolation is limited.

Clinical Application

If summarized without reservation, these results argue for clinical attention to minimizing noise in voice production, whether from an extraneous source or as a component of quality. They provide little guidance, however, with respect to goals for mean frequency and intensity levels or their variability. For speech parameters, relatively consistent encouragement exists for faster rates, limited pause, and, in most cases, higher intelligibility/articulatory accuracy to increase overall performance, particularly for ES speakers. Further evidence shows that attention needs to be paid to phonemic error on consonants, particularly pressure phonemes, with emphasis on the voiceless cognates (typically heard as voiced). No clear direction emerges for consideration of releasing versus arresting positions within syllables, at least not exclusive of manner of production.

As before, restraints to interpretation qualify clinical application. The most fundamental of these limitations results from the research designs used to identify distinguishing voice/speech characteristics. Almost without exception, these studies divided speakers according to proficiency/preference levels, and then compared features in their speech. This research format can legitimately identify presence or absence of sample differences; however, it neither confirms nor denies their influence on the original composite performance ratings. Isolation of critical components requires direct manipulation of the feature of interest with proficiency/preference as the dependent measure. Of significance, also, is the between-subject nature of these studies. As stated before, the clinical situation represents a within-subject design. This difference is particularly relevant given that certain characteristics may differ across individuals but may not be manipulable within the individual, or may be manipulable only at the risk of negatively affecting other voice/speech components.

Issues of representativeness are again relevant here. In many cases, the restricted number of speakers, and/or the limited difference in performance of speakers, precludes identification of discriminating variables. In addition, in some instances the samples used to determine the overall performance levels of the speakers were not the same as those used to measure the variable(s) of interest. Consequently, the degree of correlation between the selected feature(s) and a given skill level may simply reflect the similarity/dissimilarity in the samples used. The sample generated could even be at risk independently, considering issues in representativeness, as discussed in the preceding section.

Procedural variables are again possible influences in these data outcomes. Their impact cannot be verified, however, because none of the literature included direct comparison of alternative procedures and no two studies were sufficiently similar in other respects to allow comparison of results. Reliance on physical measures, as opposed to perceptual impressions, may restrict the influence of procedural variations in studies of voice/speech features; however, it still would be prudent to assume some impact.

Even the studies of phonemic error patterns are suspect as guides in treatment programs. Although the research designs are less at issue, concerns regarding speaker/sample representativeness are still legitimate. Applicability is at risk, also, since the errors identified may represent inherent limits of the population and, as such, may not be amenable to change.

Given the limited scope of this literature and the associated reservations, little guidance seems available for identifying subgoals universal to alaryngeal speech training. Again, the clinician could acquire data specific to the individual client, manipulating select variables and measuring their impact on composite performance; however, only a portion of the voice/speech characteristics are open to a priori evaluation, that is, before the investment of training time. Consequently, some other supplemental means is needed to structure therapy. In this case, reconsideration of the literature, despite its limits, could be helpful.

Broadly interpreted, there is some suggestion in the literature that critical features are both predictable and generally common across speech types. For example, the data on alaryngeal voice/speech characteristics offer the expected support for increased intelligibility and increased naturalness/normalcy. Furthermore, phonemic error patterns seem reasonable in light of aperiodic sound/voice sources and altered mechanisms for generating oral pressure. If this type of reasoned approach is sufficient, general knowledge of the components of the speech product could be used to structure a training program (see Figure 8.2). Obviously, the process begins by establishing the basic mechanics of sound production for a particular speech type and extends into initial attention to timing and duration. Other aspects of sound control may be directly manipulated with an AL or deferred in ES/TE speech under the assumption that they are minimally modifiable or will optimize spontaneously with continued use. Although last in the figure, potential distractors also are addressed in this initial training to avoid unacceptable patterns. Beyond this stage, emphasis shifts to factors affecting intelligibility, whether directly (e.g., oral pressure) or indirectly (e.g., rate), given the impact on functionality. Components of naturalness, then, would be last in order.

Regardless of the means by which training objectives are identified and prioritized, subsequent evaluation is still appropriate to confirm their impact on composite speech performance. Again, consideration of qualifiers to the literature interpretation provides some guidance.

1. Corroborate changes in components with physical measures where possible; do not rely on perceptual impressions.

2. Control changes in parameters other than the one intended, or at least monitor concomitant effects.
3. Ideally, use the same speech samples both for verification of the feature change and for estimation of the impact on composite performance.
4. As before, be sensitive to issues of representativeness of the data, considering both the samples used and the measures applied.

Identification of features critical to a client's voice/speech product, whether established by deduction or direct evaluation, isolates the general subgoals of therapy. However, this selection process may not lead directly to treatment instructions or procedures. In many cases, it still will be necessary to identify the processes required to accomplish these changes, for example, reducing effort to achieve reduced stoma noise or increasing oral pressure to assist recognition of voiceless phonemes.

TERMINATION LEVEL

Decision Guidelines

The final critical question in alaryngeal speech treatment is when to terminate treatment. Basic to this decision is the choice of the standard against which performance is evaluated. Unfortunately, choosing the referent and criterion is not simple. This section is not sufficient to resolve these issues, but it should amplify the factors involved.

Decisions concerning termination could be based on criteria developed from normative referenced measures where performance of the client is evaluated against that of a representative population. However, this standard presents a problem in alaryngeal speech training. Given the specialized nature of the population and the processes involved, measurement against normal (laryngeal) speakers seems unrealistic. Even if the comparative population is other alaryngeal speakers, selection of the criterion level presents a particular dilemma given the heterogeneity among clients. If the upper end of the performance spectrum is identified as the standard, optimal achievement is encouraged for all but will be accomplished by only a few. If "average" behavior is used as the goal, then a greater number will be successful but some speakers will be limited to less than their potential best.

Termination also could be based on criterion referenced measures where client performance is evaluated against a standard reflecting expected needs. This option might minimize some problems inherent to population comparisons but still leaves the issue of the actual criterion unresolved. If data were available describing minimal levels necessary for satisfactory speech, then at least the earliest point at which termination would be tolerable could be identified. Some clients still might develop short of potential, but functionality would be assured.

Ideally, some mutual consideration of individual potential and minimal requirements seems to be needed. If performance can exceed functional levels, training beyond the minimum might be considered negotiable, although admittedly, few clinicians seem particularly tolerant of an intentionally restricted outcome. However, this alternative raises the additional need for estimation of client potential.

Beyond consideration of the performance criterion for termination, one other comment, although obvious to all clinicians, bears repeating: skill acquisition does not guarantee skill utilization. As such, judgments of speech proficiency are incomplete as an index of success. Some part of the ongoing and terminal evaluation must address the client's tolerance of the speech product/process and willingness to use it. Considering these dual factors, the optimal outcome of alaryngeal speech rehabilitation would be unlimited use of unlimited speech.

This counterbalance of proficiency and utilization in termination decisions can be displayed in a schematic (Figure 8.3). Skill level (proficiency) is represented by the horizontal axis and is measured in degree. Skill use is represented by the vertical axis and is measured as frequency. The intersection of the two scales might be viewed as the point at which minimally functional speech is available for necessary communication. For a particular client, points predicting potential skill level and opportunities for skill use would be identified and marked on their respective axes. The cell outlined by extending these points from the axes would represent a range of acceptable levels for termination, with the minimum (A) identified by the intersection of the original scales (functional/necessary) and the maximum (B) identified by the intersection of the optimal predicted performance. Across clients, not only would the cell encompassing acceptable terminal levels differ, but even the intersection point identifying functional/necessary levels could alter. The realized performance would, of course, be specific to the individual.

This schema may be a fair representation of the decision process for termination and may even serve to identify treatment needs prior to termination (e.g., increase proficiency vs. increase utilization). However, it introduces even additional needs for definition with respect to skill utilization. Not only must total scale length be established for skill use, but determination of "necessary" levels must be described. As with skill level, maximum opportunity for utilization (potential) also must be estimated.

If these issues in establishing terminal goals could be resolved, then the application of composite performance measures in this decision

SKILL USE

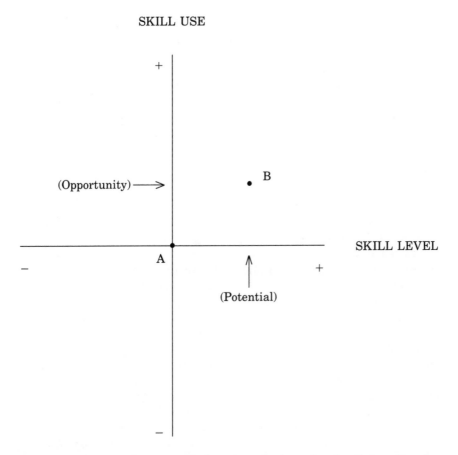

Figure 8.3. Termination points for alaryngeal speech training based on dual consideration of skill level and skill use. A = minimum acceptable outcome. B = maximum expected outcome.

process is clear. Perceptual judgments of proficiency/preference are generated and the values transferred to the skill level axis. Measurement procedures are identical to those used for other treatment questions; it is the criterion that remains debatable. If literature were available describing at least minimally necessary performance levels, then part of the problem would be resolved. Estimation of potential would still be required but might be manageable through careful assessment of the prerequisites for the various speech types.

Literature Review

Unfortunately, the literature offers little that is applicable to the decision regarding termination. As such, detailed review does not seem warranted. Normative referenced standards could be extrapolated from existing studies describing laryngeal or alaryngeal speaker groups; however, the question of suitability of imposing these performance levels as criteria still exists. No reports are available that allow extrapolation of criterion referenced measures. Even if attempts had been made to describe minimal performance needs, it is unlikely that the data would prove applicable to the individual given the multiple factors that affect "functionality."

Clinical Application

Since no literature exists to safely guide termination decisions, the clinician is left with the problem of designating the standard for composite performance for the client. No alternative may prove totally satisfactory, but awareness of the risks involved minimizes the potential complications. Alternatives range from imposing the most stringent performance criterion to employing none at all.

For one option, maximum or optimal standards can be established using normative data based either on laryngeal or superior alaryngeal speech. As a second choice, criterion-referenced objectives can be defined from estimates of client potential or communication needs. As a final option, a terminal goal can remain unstated, relying only on evidence of continued progress. The particular goal chosen requires weighing the effects on the efficiency of treatment against the influence on the outcome of treatment. However, if the prerequisites to training have been carefully considered, the result should be at least minimally satisfactory.

Issues in skill utilization remain, however, with one of the major problems being acquisition of the data base. The clinician rarely has direct knowledge of a client's speech needs or reactions in communication settings. In most cases, clients can be encouraged to provide realistic assessments of their speech opportunities, including descriptions of relative importance. Clearly, little exact commonality will occur across clients, mandating separate criteria for each. Despite this potentially cumbersome task, evaluation of skill utilization is a necessary complement to assessment of skill level if a satisfactory treatment outcome is to be assured.

Obviously, the factors involved in termination decisions are multiple and not well defined, particularly with reference to the criteria to be applied. Regardless, it is crucial that the comparative measures used in this terminal assessment meet stringent criteria for accuracy/

applicability for the particular client. Consequently, the issues raised in the preceding sections are equally relevant for the measures of both skill level and skill use, with the primary concern being representativeness of the data. Given the vital nature of this final step in the decision sequence, these measures should be acquired with exceptional care.

SUMMARY

The intent of this chapter was to highlight the role of perceptual judgments of proficiency/preference in alaryngeal speech training. Although not sufficient in themselves, they do contribute to the data needed for treatment decisions. Specifically, these measures are applicable in comparisons of the relative merits of the speech alternatives, in isolation of critical subgoals, and in determination of program success.

Consideration also was given to literature based on these composite performance measures to determine applicability to these decision processes. Unfortunately, the studies reviewed were of limited utility in this context. Questions were raised about both the relevance of the designs to the clinical setting and the representativeness of the data with respect to individual performance.

Despite the lack of immediately applicable literature, other guidelines are available for organizing treatment. In large part, it appears that basic knowledge of the population and the processes involved can provide substantial structure. However, information also is needed that is descriptive of the individual. Perceptual judgments of proficiency/preference can assist with this task; however, systematic data gathering and sensitivity in data interpretation are needed, given their critical role in treatment.

REFERENCES

Anderson, R. (1986). *Consistency within speaker and within instrument in measures of artificial larynx speech.* Unpublished master's thesis, University of Kansas, Lawrence, KS.

Bennett, S., & Weinberg, B. (1973). Acceptability ratings of normal, esophageal, and artificial larynx speech. *Journal of Speech and Hearing Research, 16,* 608–615.

Berlin, C. I. (1963). Clinical measurement of esophageal speech: I. Methodology and curves of skill acquisition. *Journal of Speech and Hearing Disorders, 28,* 42–51.

Berlin, C. I. (1965). Clinical measurement of esophageal speech: III. Performance of nonbiased groups. *Journal of Speech and Hearing Disorders, 30,* 174–183.

Blom, E., Singer, M., & Hamaker, R. (1986). A prospective study of tracheoesophageal speech. *Archives of Otolaryngology, Head and Neck Surgery, 112,* 440–447.

Cady, B. (1981). *Phonemic intelligibility in artificial larynx speech.* Unpublished doctoral dissertation, University of Kansas, Lawrence, KS.

Clark, J. G. (1985). Alaryngeal speech intelligibility and the older listener. *Journal of Speech and Hearing Disorders, 50,* 60–65.

Clark, J. G., & Stemple, J. C. (1982). Assessment of three modes of alaryngeal speech with a Synthetic Sentence Identification (SSI) task in varying message-to-competition ratios. *Journal of Speech and Hearing Research, 25,* 333–338.

Creech, J. B. (1966). Evaluating esophageal speech. *Journal of the Speech and Hearing Association of Virginia, 7,* 13–19.

Crouse, G. P. (1962). *An experimental study of esophageal and artificial larynx speech.* Unpublished master's thesis, Emory University, Atlanta, GA.

Doyle, P. C., Danhauer, J. L., & Reed, C. G. (1988). Listeners' perceptions of consonants produced by esophageal and tracheoesophageal talkers. *Journal of Speech and Hearing Disorders, 53,* 400–407.

Doyle, P. C., & Haaf, R. G. (1987). *Pre- and post-vocalic consonant intelligibility in tracheoesophageal speakers.* Paper presented at the American Speech–Language–Hearing Association National Convention, New Orleans, LA.

Filter, M. D., & Hyman, M. (1975). Relationship of acoustic parameters and perceptual ratings of esophageal speech. *Perceptual and Motor Skills, 40,* 63–68.

Goldstein, L. P. (1978). Listener judgments of artificial larynx speech. In S. J. Salmon & L. P. Goldstein (Eds.), *The artificial larynx handbook* (pp. 27–33). New York: Grune & Stratton.

Goldstein, L. P., Rothman, H. B., & Merwin, G. E. (1984). *Intrasubject comparisons of artificial larynx and tracheoesophageal puncture speech.* Poster session, American Speech–Language–Hearing Association National Convention, San Francisco, CA.

Golper, L. C., & Rau, M. T. (1978). *Laryngectomees who use esophageal speech and electrolarynx: A clinical study.* Paper presented at the American Speech–Language–Hearing Association National Convention, San Francisco, CA.

Goshorn, E. L., & Schinsky, L. E. (1976). *The intelligibility of three electrolarynges.* Paper presented at the American Speech–Language–Hearing Association National Convention, Houston, TX.

Green, G., & Hults, M. (1982). Preferences for three types of alaryngeal speech. *Journal of Speech and Hearing Disorders, 47,* 141–145.

Henley-Cohn, J. L., Hausfeld, J. N., & Jakubcsak, G. (1984). Artificial larynx prosthesis: Comparative clinical evaluation. *Laryngoscope, 94,* 43–45.

Hoops, H. R., & Guzek, T. J. (1974). The relationship of rate and phrasing to esophageal speech proficiency. *Archives of Otolaryngology, 100,* 190–193.

Hoops, H. R., & Noll, J. D. (1969). Relationship of selected acoustic variables to judgments of esophageal speech. *Journal of Communication Disorders, 2,* 1–13.

Horii, Y., & Weinberg, B. (1975). Intelligibility characteristics of superior esophageal speech presented under various levels of masking noise. *Journal of Speech and Hearing Research, 18,* 413–419.

Hyman, M. (1955). An experimental study of artificial larynx and esophageal speech. *Journal of Speech and Hearing Disorders, 20,* 291–299.

Kalb, M. B., & Carpenter, M. A. (1981). Individual speaker influence on relative intelligibility of esophageal and artificial larynx speech. *Journal of Speech and Hearing Disorders, 46,* 77–80.

Kelly, D. (1979). The effects of restricting parameters of the speech excitation function of an electronic larynx: A pilot study. In R. L. Keith & F. L. Darley (Eds.), *Laryngectomee rehabilitation* (pp. 521–533). Austin, TX: PRO-ED.

McCroskey, R. L., & Mulligan, M. (1963). The relative intelligibility of esophageal speech and artificial-larynx speech. *Journal of Speech and Hearing Disorders, 29*, 37–41.

Rothman, H. B. (1978). Analyzing artificial electronic speech. In S. J. Salmon & L. P. Goldstein (Eds.), *The artificial larynx handbook* (pp. 87–111). New York: Grune & Stratton.

Sacco, P. R., Mann, M. B., & Schultz, M. C. (1967). Perceptual confusions among selected phonemes in esophageal speech. *Journal of the Indiana Speech and Hearing Association, 26*, 19–33.

Shames, G. H., Font, J., & Matthews, J. (1963). Factors related to speech proficiency of the laryngectomized. *Journal of Speech and Hearing Disorders, 29*, 273–287.

Shipp, T. (1967). Frequency, duration, and perceptual measures in relation to judgments of alaryngeal speech acceptability. *Journal of Speech and Hearing Research, 10*, 417–427.

Stalker, J. L., Hawk, A. M., & Smaldino, J. J. (1982). The intelligibility and acceptability of speech produced by five different electronic artificial larynx devices. *Journal of Communications Disorders, 15*, 299–307.

Trudeau, M. D. (1987). A comparison of the speech acceptability of good and excellent esophageal and tracheoesophageal speakers. *Journal of Communication Disorders, 20*, 41–49.

Weiss, M. S., & Basili, A. G. (1985). Electrolaryngeal speech produced by laryngectomized subjects: Perceptual characteristics. *Journal of Speech and Hearing Research, 28*, 294–300.

Weiss, M. S., Yeni-Komshian, G. H., & Heinz, J. M. (1979). Acoustical and perceptual characteristics of speech produced with an electronic artificial larynx. *Journal of the Acoustical Society of America, 65*, 1298–1308.

Wetmore, S. J., Krueger, K., & Wesson, K. (1981). The Singer–Blom speech rehabilitation procedure. *The Laryngoscope, 91*, 1109–1116.

Williams, S. E., & Watson, J. B. (1984). *Variations in ratings of speaking proficiencies across three laryngectomee groups.* Paper presented at the American Speech–Language–Hearing Association National Convention, San Francisco, CA.

Zwitman, D. H., & Disinger, R. S. (1975). Experimental modification of the Western Electric #5 electrolarynx to a mouth-type instrument. *Journal of Speech and Hearing Disorders, 40*, 35–39.

Zwitman, D. H., Knorr, S. G., & Sonderman, J. C. (1978). Development and testing for an intraoral electrolarynx for laryngectomy patients. *Journal of Speech and Hearing Disorders, 54*, 263–269.

CHAPTER 9

Failure in Acquiring Esophageal Speech

Stuart I. Gilmore

> *Gilmore suggests that understanding the reasons for failure to acquire esophageal speech is essential to successful treatment of the alaryngeal speaker. He contends that knowledge of physical, social, occupational, and psychological causes of failure will help the clinician design a therapy program to prevent patterns of speech failure from becoming firmly entrenched.*

Study Questions

1. *Consider Mr. Malavoz who has been in speech therapy for 3 months following laryngectomy but is able to produce only a few inconsistent vowels or one-syllable words. How will you determine what physical problems are contributing to his failure? How should they be managed? What should be done if for some reason they cannot be managed medically? Why?*

2. *How might the factors affecting the acquisition of esophageal speech also affect the acquisition of artificial larynx speech or tracheoesophageal (puncture) speech? How might having failed to learn esophageal voice affect acquisition of another form of alaryngeal speech?*

3. *Indicate one physical, one social, one occupational, and one psychological problem that you think might impede speech acquisition in a given client. Suggest how these problems might be anticipated, averted, or managed in a preventive program. How will you determine whether your preventive programs are effective?*

In this chapter, *esophageal speech* refers to a laryngectomized individual's ability to (a) inflate the esophagus by means of inhalation or injection, (b) use the air trapped in the esophagus to generate esophageal tone at the pharyngoesophageal junction (also called the pharyngoesophageal, or PE, segment), and (c) use the esophageal voice to generate esophageal speech that is sufficiently intelligible, fluent, and comfortable to support resumption of the communication functions assumed prior to laryngectomy.

Understanding what constitutes and contributes to failure to acquire esophageal speech is as important to the speech clinician as understanding how esophageal speech is taught. That importance is evidenced by continuing concerns expressed by clients, families, and clinicians; by the extent of the clinical and research literature dealing with problems of speech acquisition; and by recent reports suggesting increasing failure rates.

This chapter is intended to clarify the nature and extent of esophageal speech failure, the factors that can result in failure, and considerations for their management.

Reports of successful esophageal speech acquisition vary from 13% to 74% in the extended literature, and from 26% to 68%, with an average of 50%, in the last decade. Concern has been generated by the findings of Gates and his associates, who concluded from their data that the potential for acquiring esophageal speech and achieving rehabilitation goals is considerably less than has been reported in the past (Gates & Hearne, 1982; Gates, Ryan, Cantu, & Hearne, 1982; Gates, Ryan, Cooper, et al., 1982; Gates, Ryan, & Lauder, 1982). Whereas 62% of their 40 retrospectively studied subjects had acquired esophageal speech, only 26% of the 47 prospectively studied subjects used esophageal speech for daily communication. The increased frequency of failure in the prospective group was attributed to increases in patient age, tumor advancement, and number and intensiveness of therapeutic modalities used (surgery, radiotherapy, chemotherapy) in patients needing total laryngectomy.

Concern regarding failure has also been generated by research and clinical observations that many who use esophageal speech do so imperfectly, or with need to rely on an artificial larynx or writing to augment communication.

The variability of success rates probably reflects many factors, including differences in treatment modalities used, or in specific procedures within a given modality, in programs of management, and in the criteria used to determine speech success. An implicit assumption made by most investigators, writers, and clinicians appears to have been that success depended, at least partially, upon the extent to which the speaker used esophageal speech. "Successful" speakers relied solely upon esophageal speech, and were then subclassified as superior speakers, or as less than superior but "functional" esophageal speakers. "Failures" included those speakers unable to rely on esophageal speech, particularly those depending solely on artificial larynx speech.

Only occasionally and relatively recently has the literature suggested that failure should be appraised as the degree of restriction in *oral* communication rather than in standard *esophageal communication.* In this case, failure would entail the inability to use either esophageal or artificial larynx speech, and consequently would deprive the individual of the spontaneity and freedom of oral communication, including use of the telephone. (Sadly, Volin [1980] found speechlessness in 40% of his 59 subjects.) Conversely, success would be determined by the extent to which a speaker could accomplish his or her intents orally, regardless of speech mode, and ratings would reflect or classify speakers as being superior, functional, nonfunctional, or nonspeakers. The findings of Gates and colleagues suggest that we need to look toward this model of speech rehabilitation at the same time that we pursue understanding why people fail to learn esophageal speech (Gates & Hearne, 1982; Gates, Ryan, Cantu, & Hearne, 1982; Gates, Ryan, Cooper, et al., 1982; Gates, Ryan, & Lauder, 1982).

FACTORS THAT CAN IMPEDE ACQUISITION OF ESOPHAGEAL SPEECH

The remainder of this chapter examines the many variables that can impede or preclude esophageal speech acquisition. They are discussed under six categories of factors, with recognition that these categories generally coexist and interact: physical, social, occupational, psychological, training, and idiopathic. The objective is to clarify these factors, including considerations for the evaluation and management of the physical factors. Appreciation of how failure can occur should ultimately increase the level and rate of client success and consequently of clinician satisfaction.

Physical Factors

Included in the physical factors category are deficits of speech organ configuration, motor speech function, and/or sensation (auditory, tactile, and movement), often referred to as organic deficits. These may be congenital or acquired conditions predating the laryngectomy, age-related conditions (the approximate mean age of the laryngectomized population is 55 years), or surgical residuals, such as glossopharyngeal nerve damage following radical neck dissection or an "inadequately reconstructed" neoglottis.

Structural and physiological factors can impair esophageal speech acquisition both indirectly and directly. Indirectly, they act in two ways: by absorbing energies that could otherwise be directed toward speech development, and by restricting the need, opportunity, and desire to communicate. Indirect factors involve an array of physical disorders, including but not restricted to:

- Changes in sensation (notably smell and taste), biological functions (respiration, coughing—the presence of a stoma), deglutition, and digestion.
- Physical limitations, particularly after radical neck dissection or radiotherapy, for example, shoulder and neck dysfunctions and discomfort, and diminished salivation.
- Problems associated with illness, for example, respiratory problems related to having smoked, and possibly alcohol abuse.
- Problems associated with aging, including degenerative diseases, hearing loss, cardiovascular and cerebrovascular disorders, senility, and the possible negative effects of medications taken for these disorders.
- Problems associated with recurrent or additional cancers.

Physical factors that directly hamper esophageal speech development consist of deficits that impede the learning and refinement of speech motor acts designed to rectify or compensate for the loss of the pulmonary air supply and the laryngeal source tone in speech production. Specifically, physical deficits prevent or restrict one or more of the following goals of speech training: (a) trapping air in the esophagus; (b) producing and regulating esophageal tone (quality, pitch, loudness, duration, and prosodic elements); and (c) producing readily intelligible and aesthetic connected speech (articulating, notably differentiating voiced–voiceless–nasal homologues, phrasing, stressing, and eliminating or minimizing stomal masking noise and visible or audible distracters). Clinically the acquisition and refinement of esophageal voice appears to be the major problem area and, consequently, the major source of failure to develop esophageal speech. For this reason, factors directly affecting esophageal voice development, and their management, are discussed next.

Failure to Acquire Esophageal Voice. Two propositions underlie this section. First, consistent and controlled esophageal *voice* is the primary objective when teaching esophageal *speech*, both in its importance for speech acquisition and in its place in the sequence of training objectives. Second, physical problems constitute a major source of failure to acquire esophageal voice. Critical problems, and eventual failure, occur more frequently when initiating esophageal voice training than when refining voice or articulation. (The reader is referred to chapters

3 and 4 for detailed discussions of esophageal speech training goals and procedures.)

The vulnerability of patients during the early stages of training probably reflects both psychological and physical factors. Psychologically, the patient's early postsurgical impressions of the nature and extent of loss generate immense stress, depression, and defensive retreat. These reactions are not conducive to learning and practicing new speech skills. Additionally, the early goals of trapping air in the esophagus and producing a reliable esophageal tone are particularly vulnerable to structural and physiological disorders. Moreover, these initial goals are prerequisites for the refinement of duration, quality, prosody, and articulation, which should eventually establish both esophageal speech intelligibility and listener attention. It is critical that speech clinicians understand the physical deterrents to early speech development.

The objective of this section is to clarify physical problems underlying failure to acquire esophageal voice. Included are (a) the requisites for trapping air in the esophagus and for producing esophageal tone; (b) the structural, neuromotor, and sensory disorders compromising those requisites, and their symptoms; and (c) suggested assessment and treatment modalities. These problems and their management are summarized in Table 9.1. Additionally, the reasons for failure after voice acquisition will be discussed briefly.

Trapping Air in the Esophagus. Trapping air in the esophagus to power esophageal speech requires two abilities: the ability to create a pressure differential above and below the PE segment, and the ability to inflate the esophagus. The literature and clinical experience indicate that injection is the major method used by esophageal speakers to charge the esophagus with air. To inject, pharyngeal pressure must exceed esophageal pressure to a degree sufficient to overcome PE segment resistance (see Figure 9.1). The injector must be able both to seal the oropharyngeal cavities so that the air contained therein *can* be compressed, and to decrease cavity volume to accomplish compression. Volume reduction/compression results primarily from lingual action, and possibly from labial and pharyngeal action.

Inflating the esophagus with air also requires two abilities: the ability to transport oropharyngeal air inferiorly through the PE segment, and the ability to contain the injected air in the upper esophagus for phonatory use.

Air transport problems are generally due to excessive resistance at the esophageal port, reflecting either hypopharyngeal obstructions (pouches or diverticuli, and strictures) or PE segment tension problems (inability to relax the sphincter). Pouches and diverticuli are abnormal, circumscribed sacs or forward bulgings occurring high (just below the

TABLE 9.1
Failure to Develop Esophageal Voice: Problems and Their Management

	Problem			Management
Incapacity	Disorder	Signs	Assessment	Treatment
I. Trapping Air in the Esophagus A. Inability to seal cavity 1. at nasopharyngeal port	1. Structural: palatal configuration and length 2. Neuromotor: velopharyngeal paresis 3. Sensory: oral anesthesia; hearing loss	Cleft palate, restricted palatopharyngeal movement, nasal regurgitation; difficulty following directions	Cine or videofluoroscopy (see Perry, 1983, p. 184, for brief description of procedure); nasendoscopy; audiologic evaluation	1. Prosthetic: palatal appliance (bulb, lift); nares occluding appliance 2. Surgical: palatoplasty, pharyngoplasty (pharyngeal flap, implant) 3. Speech: if not physically remediable, alternatives are inhalation technique, artificial larynx, tracheoesophageal puncture/fistulization (TEP speech); may require therapy for articulation and/or hypernasality
2. at oral port (lips, tongue)	1. Structural: glossectomy mandibulectomy, maxillectomy 2. Neuromotor: labial or lingual paresis (latter can follow radical neck dissection) 3. Sensory: oral/lingual anesthesia (can follow radical neck dissection); hearing loss	Drooping lip, drooling, inability to close lips or elevate lower lip or tongue, eating and drinking difficulties, misarticulated labial and/or lingual sounds; complaints of sensation loss; difficulty following directions	Observation of eating, drinking, smiling, speaking; cine or videofluoroscopy; audiologic evaluation	1. Prosthetic: palatal drop appliance; dental appliance (or more extensive, if required) 2. Speech: labial/lingual range–strength–precision of motion; alternatives are inhalation technique, artificial larynx, TEP, may require articulation therapy
B. Inability to compress air within the oropharyngeal cavities	As in IA2	As in IA2	As in IA2	As in IA2
C. Inability to transport air through the PE segment	1. Structural: pouches/diverticuli (see Figures 9.2 and 9.3), strictures; PE segment excessively long (see Figure 9.4), multiple segments	History of fistulae; *perhaps* difficulty swallowing, regurgitation; contrast medium puddling; pharyngeal voice (air trapped in hypopharynx is used to power a vibrator above it, compromising vocal quality, duration, and articulation—see Figure 9.11)	Cine or videofluoroscopy (barium swallow); endoscopy; manometry (see Figures 9.5 and 9.6)	1. Medical/Surgical: medication (muscle relaxants, tranquilizers); pharyngoesophageal dilation (bouginage, catheter and syringe); myotomy, mucosal revision, surgical release of stricture (may result in PE segment hypotonia). 2. Speech: with pouch/diverticuli observe effects of adjusting head posture or digital manipulation, diet or medication to reduce secretions; for PE segment hypertension reduce stress and anxiety, relaxation, biofeedback, hypnosis

Table continues

TABLE 9.1 Continued

	Problem			Management	
Incapacity	Disorder	Signs	Assessment	Treatment	

	Problem			Management	
	Disorder	Signs	Assessment	Treatment	
D. Inability to contain air within the esophagus	1. Sphincteric and gastrointestinal problems, either structural or neuromotor: hiatal hernia (controversial cause of speech failure); achalasia	Hiatus hernia: heartburn, regurgitation, sensation food sticking in throat, chest pain, "wet" voice quality. Achalasia: dysphagia, pain, regurgitation, weight loss	Gastroenterological: manometry, fluoroscopy, endoscopy	1. Medical/Surgical: anti-reflex herniaplasty; esophagocardiomyotomy for achalasia	
II. Producing Esophageal Tone					
A. Insufficient PE segment resistance for phonation (hypotonicity)	1. Structural: lack of constricting muscle fibers (see Figures 9.7 and 9.8, which contrast adequate and hypotonic PE segments), e.g. following laryngopharyngoesophagectomy, gastric pull-up, colon transplant, tissue flaps (see Figures 9.9 and 9.10) 2. Neuromotor: surgically compromised hypopharyngeal innervation	Absent peristalsis during barium swallow (no swallow problems); weak voice; "bubbly" voice due to gastric contents proximity; pharyngeal voice (see Figures 9.11 and 9.12)	Cine or videofluoroscopy	1. Surgical: sternomastoid muscle swing 2. Speech: adjusting head posture or applying digital pressure (release to inject and press to phonate) to narrow the PE segment and/or prevent bulging or ballooning by introducing resistance anterior to the neoglottis (see Figures 9.11 and 9.12); applying a pressure band around the neck (see Figure 9.13); amplification (see Figure 9.14)	
B. Excessive PE segment resistance (hypertonicity, spasm)	1. Structural: excessively long or multiple PE segment; recurrent cancer 2. Neuromotor: reflexive response to esophageal inflation (possibly "normal")	Absent or inconsistent esophageal sound, even following esophageal inflation (validate by audible klunks on injection or clicks on inhalation, tactile clues, patient report of chest fullness, and/or by air insufflation testing); strictures absent on scoping or X-ray, but may demonstrate multiple or excessively long PE segment; may demonstrate esophageal distension due to air intake without the ability to expel it	Air insufflation test, possibly in association with pharyngeal plexus nerve block and cine or videofluoroscopy	1. Surgical/Medical: as in IC; myotomy from tongue base downward, including medial and inferior constrictors and cricopharyngeus; neurectomy (currently being explored experimentally) 2. Speech: as in IC, plus clinical techniques used to reduce stuttering blocks or laryngeal hyperfunction	

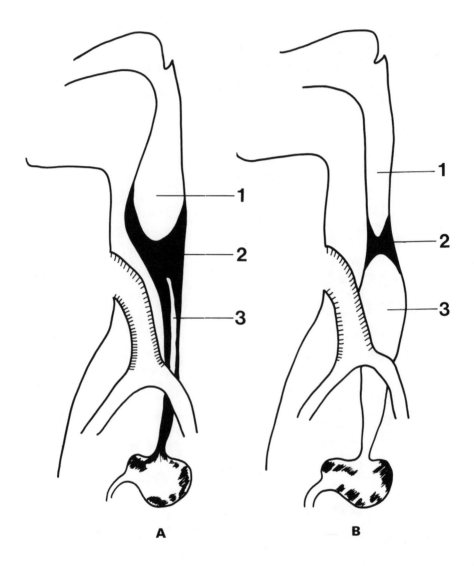

Figure 9.1. Schematic diagram showing relative air pressures in the new vocal tract. (A) Hypopharyngeal pressure elevated prior to injection. (B) Esophageal pressure elevated on initiating phonation. 1 = hypopharynx; 2 = pharyngoesophageal segment; 3 = esophagus.

tongue base at the level of the hyoid bone) or low (between the PE junction and the hyoid bone) in the anterior pharyngeal wall (see Figure 9.2). Pouches are thought to reflect complications of wound healing that result in an irregular shape, or a fistula that should heal before speech therapy continues (see Figure 9.3). Strictures are narrowings (scarring, fibrosis), other than the PE segment, that are located between the oropharynx and the esophagus. Three types occur: permanent strictures, which do not distend, even during swallowing; pseudostrictures, or bulgings of posterior pharyngeal wall into the hypopharyngeal lumen; and voluntary contractions, which are visible only on phonation and not during injection, swallowing, or rest (Simpson, Smith, & Gordon, 1972). Recent writings suggest that pseudostrictures and voluntary contractions may actually be signs of PE segment hypertonicity and spasm, discussed later.

Resistance to air transport can also reflect inability to relax the PE segment. In laryngeal individuals, the PE segment is usually closed, and opens only after it is relaxed. Generally, relaxation occurs reflexively during swallowing, when pharyngeal pressure is elevated by the pumping action of the oral floor. Inflating the esophagus requires the ability to relax the PE segment voluntarily, at least to the point at which air pressure differentials above and below the segment can overcome its resistance to airflow.

Physical problems that can impair esophageal inflation can, and often do, impair esophageal phonation. Figures 9.4 and 9.5 show the X-ray and manometric tracing of a patient demonstrating excessive resistance to esophageal inflation, and a consequent inability to trap air or to produce esophageal voice. Figure 9.6 demonstrates the increase in PE segment tension and decrease in air input (reduced gastric air bubble size) in a group of patients who were unable to acquire esophageal speech compared with a group having excellent esophageal voices. PE segment difficulties are explored more fully in the section on producing esophageal tone.

Inability to contain air in the esophagus for phonatory use is thought to be related to cardiac (distal) sphincter incompetence and gastro-esophageal problems. The distal sphincter, which separates the stomach and esophagus, is normally closed except to permit food, liquid, or airflow in either direction, as needed. Although controversial, its function, and consequently air containment for esophageal voice, may be compromised by hiatal (distal sphincter) hernia or achalasia (a sphincteric–lower esophageal muscle incoordination disorder of possible neurogenic origin).

Producing a Reliable Esophageal Tone Capable of Being Shaped into Speech. Once air is trapped in the esophagus, the next task is

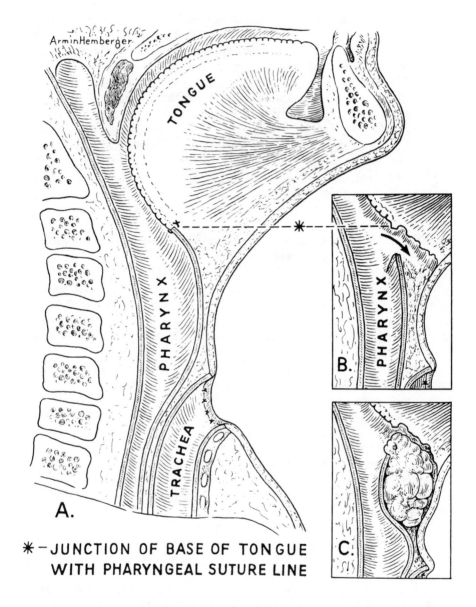

*— JUNCTION OF BASE OF TONGUE WITH PHARYNGEAL SUTURE LINE

Figure 9.2. Mechanism of development of postoperative pouch at base of tongue. The upper end of the pharyngeal suture line separates at its junction with the base of the tongue. Oral secretions and ingesta may enter this defect and result in a permanent pouch, as shown. If the secretions reach the skin surface, a fistula is formed. From "The Pharynx After Laryngectomy: Changes in Its Structure and Function" by J. A. Kirchner, J. H. Scatliff, F. L. Dey, and D. P. Shedd, 1963, *The Laryngoscope, 73,* p. 25. Copyright 1963 by the Laryngoscope Company. Reprinted by permission.

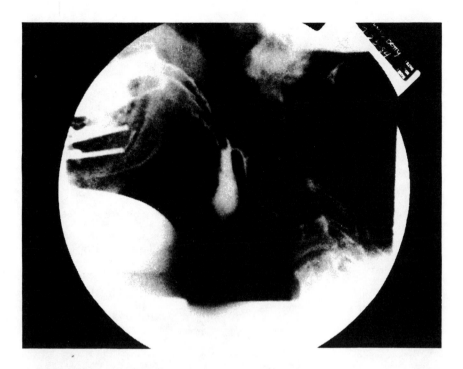

Figure 9.3. X-ray demonstrating a pouch filled with barium anterior to the pharyngo-esophageal segment after the barium swallow is completed. From "Clinical considerations in management of the laryngectomee" by D. D. Fox, in *Laryngectomee Rehabilitation* (2nd ed., p. 387) by R. L. Keith and F. L. Darley (Eds.), 1986, Austin, TX: PRO-ED. Copyright 1986 by PRO-ED, Inc. Reprinted by permission of PRO-ED, Inc.

esophageal phonation. This task requires expulsion of the esophageal air through a PE segment that has sufficient resistance to that airflow to generate an esophageal source tone, but not so much resistance that the tone is excessively strained, inconsistent, or unable to be generated. Moreover, when esophageal tone is shaped later in therapy into increasingly intelligible and acceptable esophageal speech, it will require a generating system that will support increased duration and prosodic variation of pitch, loudness, and duration. The critical element in successful esophageal phonation may well be the ability to regulate PE segment tension, and the major obstacles are either segment hypotonicity/flaccidity or hypertonicity/spasm.

The pharyngoesophageal segment/junction is formed by cricopharyngeal and pharyngeal constrictor muscle fibers, usually located at the

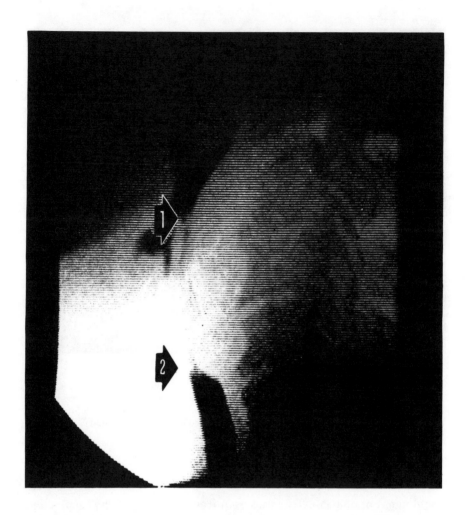

Figure 9.4. Exceptionally long (7-cm) pharyngoesophageal segment (between arrows) in a postlaryngectomy patient (E.G.) who experienced significant difficulty swallowing and inability to inflate the esophagus for voice production. From "Radiographic and manometric assessment of the patient who fails to acquire esophageal voice" by E. D. Blom, in *Laryngectomee Rehabilitation* (p. 194) by R. L. Keith and F. L. Darley (Eds.), 1979, Austin, TX: PRO-ED. Copyright 1979 by PRO-ED, Inc. Reprinted by permission of PRO-ED, Inc.

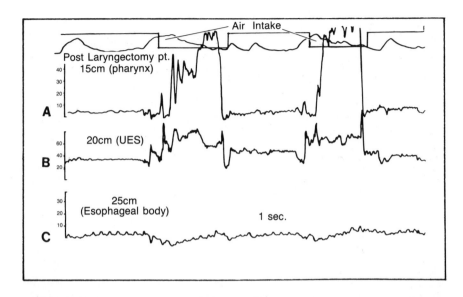

Figure 9.5. Manometric recording (mm Hg) during attempted air injection in a postlaryngectomy patient (E.G.) having an exceptionally long pharyngoesophageal (PE) segment. (A) Tracing from transducer in the pharynx. (B) PE segment. (C) Body of esophagus. Note simultaneous increase in pharyngeal and PE segment pressures during unsuccessful attempts to insufflate the esophagus. From "Radiographic and manometric assessment of the patient who fails to acquire esophageal voice" by E. D. Blom, in *Laryngectomee Rehabilitation* (p. 199) by R. L. Keith and F. L. Darley (Eds.), 1979, Austin, TX: PRO-ED. Copyright 1979 by PRO-ED, Inc. Reprinted by permission of PRO-ED, Inc.

level of the fifth or sixth cervical vertebra. The normal segment is typically seen radiographically during esophageal phonation as an esophageal narrowing occurring below a conically shaped hypopharynx and above an inflated esophagus, giving the region a characteristic hourglass configuration (see Figure 9.7).

Radiographically, the PE narrowing would appear flattened or absent in patients having hypotonic or flaccid PE segments (see Figure 9.8). Flaccid sphincters often occur following extensive surgery (laryngectomy plus esophagectomy), such as the procedures illustrated in Figures 9.9 and 9.10.

The voice produced by a hypotonic or flaccid PE segment will sound "breathy," weak in intensity, and short in duration, or may be lacking entirely. Excessively long segments, multiple segments, and pouches and strictures can also impede phonation, the latter frequently causing

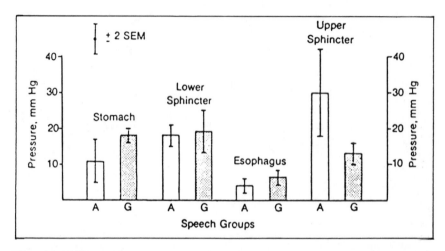

Figure 9.6. Mean pressures from stomach, lower esophageal sphincter, midesophagus, and cricopharyngeal sphincter of (A) 7 laryngectomees unable to acquire esophageal speech and (G) 8 with excellent esophageal voices. From "Esophageal Determinants of Alaryngeal Speech" by C. S. Winans, E. J. Reichbach, and W. F. Waldrop, 1974, *Archives of Otolaryngology, 98*, p. 12. Copyright 1974 by the American Medical Association. Reprinted by permission.

wet or "gurgly" vocal quality. The speech pathologist confronted with the "breathy," poorly audible voice accompanying a hypnotic/flaccid PE segment might consider digital pressure, pressure bands, or amplification to manage the problem (see Figures 9.11, 9.12, 9.13, and 9.14). When esophageal phonation is impeded by insufficient or excessive PE segment resistance, pharyngeal voice may develop in its place. Pharyngeal voice uses air stored in the pharynx to activate a vibrator composed of the tongue and the pharyngeal wall, soft palate or faucial pillars (see Figures 9.15 and 9.16). Pharyngeal voice might well occur in the patient demonstrated in Figure 9.4. It did occur in the patient demonstrated in Figure 9.8.

Pharyngoesophageal spasm has been implicated as a significant cause of failure to develop esophageal voice (Singer & Blom, 1981). Radiographically, PE spasm would be demonstrated by transient formation of a pronounced posterior pharyngeal constrictor mass protruding into the esophageal lumen, and forming an airtight barrier. McGarvey and Weinberg (1984) suggested that airtight closure may be a "normal" response to esophageal insufflation, and that the ability to produce consistent and continuous esophageal tone may actually be a sign of a

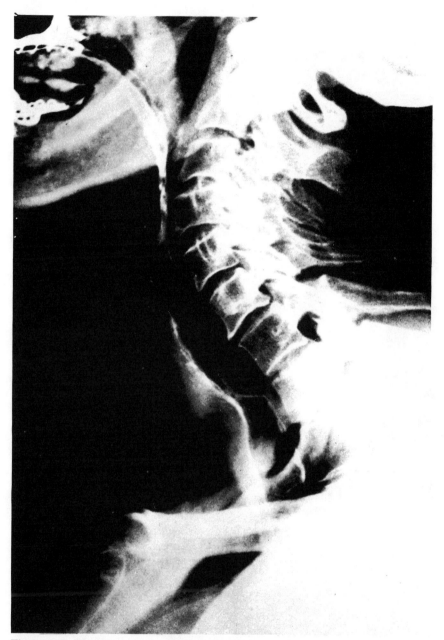

Figure 9.7. X-ray demonstrating the constricted pharyngoesophageal segment below the hypopharynx and above the inflated esophagus in a superior speaker producing the vowel /a/. From "Surgery and speech, the pseudoglottis, and respiration in total standard laryngectomy" by E. R. Finkbeiner, in *Speech Rehabilitation of the Laryngectomized* (2nd ed., p. 70) by J. C. Snidecor (Ed.), 1974, Springfield, IL: Charles C. Thomas. Copyright 1974 by Charles C. Thomas, Publisher. Reprinted by permission.

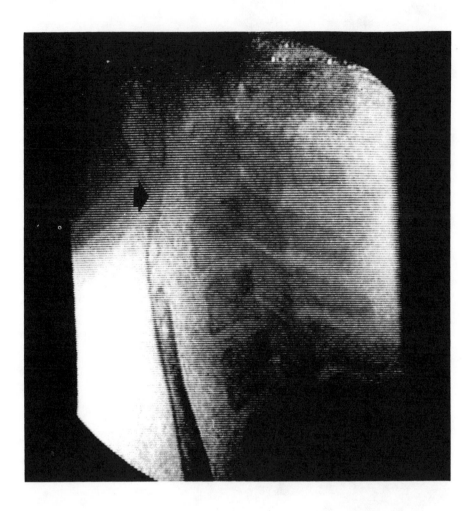

Figure 9.8. Proximal esophagus in a postlaryngectomy patient (S.B.) who developed pharyngeal rather than esophageal voice. Note the total absence of any pharyngoesophageal segment with the exception of a very slight notch (arrow). From "Radiographic and manometric assessment of the patient who fails to acquire esophageal voice" by E. D. Blom, in *Laryngectomee Rehabilitation* (p. 191) by R. L. Keith and F. L. Darley (Eds.), 1979, Austin, TX: PRO-ED. Copyright 1979 by PRO-ED, Inc. Reprinted by permission of PRO-ED, Inc.

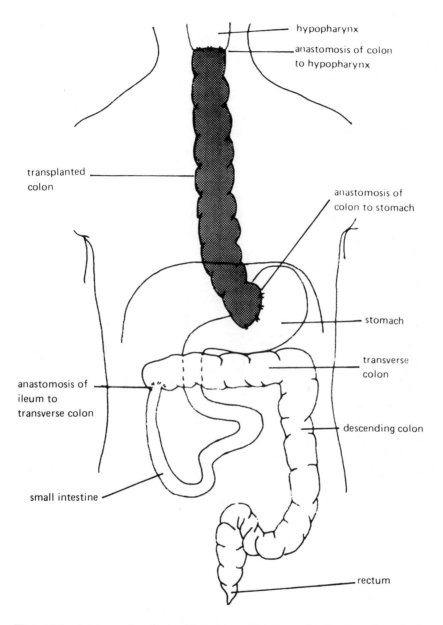

Figure 9.9. Anatomy after pharyngolaryngoesophagectomy, showing transplanted colon in position. From "Extensive surgery for post-cricoid carcinoma and subsequent vocal rehabilitation: A. Extensive surgery for post-cricoid carcinoma" by D. Ranger, in *Laryngectomy: Diagnosis to Rehabilitation* (p. 229) by Y. Edels (Ed.), Rockville, MD: Aspen. Copyright 1983 by Yvonne Edels. Reprinted by permission.

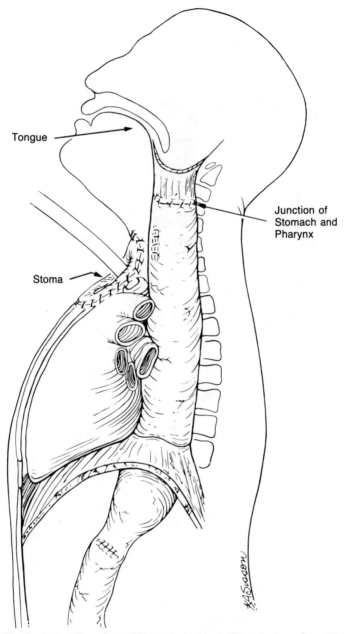

Tongue

Junction of
Stomach and
Pharynx

Stoma

Figure 9.10.   Reconstruction after total laryngectomy, esophagectomy, and gastric pull-up.
From "Extensive surgery for post-cricoid carcinoma and subsequent vocal rehabilitation:
B. Vocal rehabilitation after extensive surgery for post-cricoid carcinoma" by J. A.
Logemann, in *Laryngectomy: Diagnosis to Rehabilitation* (p. 236) by Y. Edels (Ed.), 1983,
Rockville, MD: Aspen. Copyright 1983 by Yvonne Edels. Reprinted by permission.

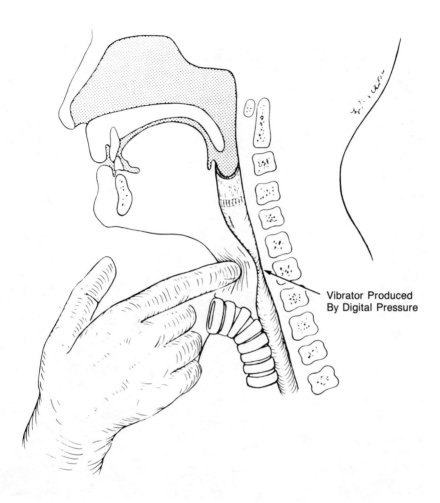

Figure 9.11. Application of digital pressure to produce a neoglottis in a patient who has had a total laryngectomy, esophagectomy, and gastric pull-up. From "Extensive surgery for post-cricoid carcinoma and subsequent vocal rehabilitation: B. Vocal rehabilitation after extensive surgery for post-cricoid carcinoma" by J. A. Logemann, in *Laryngectomy: Diagnosis to Rehabilitation* (p. 238) by Y. Edels (Ed.), 1983, London: Croom Helm. Copyright 1983 by Yvonne Edels. Reprinted by permission.

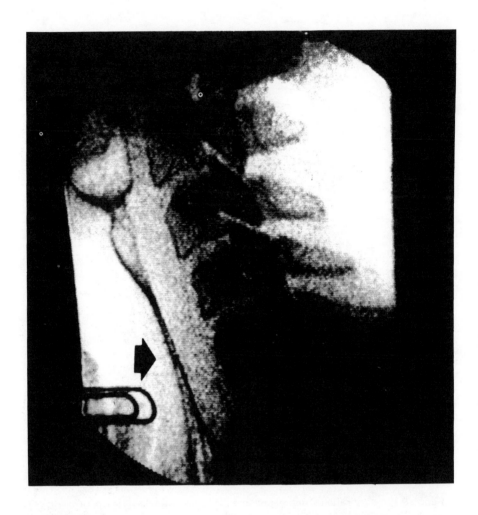

Figure 9.12. Formation of a pharyngoesophageal segment (arrow) by digital pressure against the anterior neck in a patient (S.B.). A paper clip taped to the finger is used for digital compression and serves as a location marker. From "Radiographic and manometric assessment of the patient who fails to acquire esophageal voice" by E. D. Blom, in *Laryngectomy Rehabilitation* (p. 193) by R. L. Keith and F. L. Darley (Eds.), 1979, Austin, TX: PRO-ED. Copyright 1979 by PRO-ED, Inc. Reprinted by permission of PRO-ED, Inc.

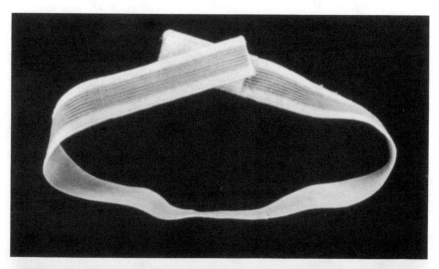

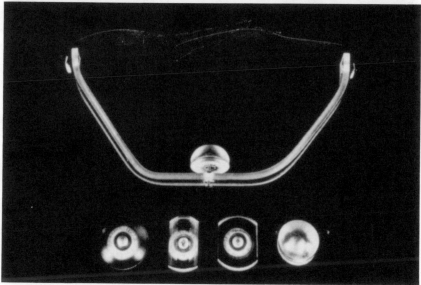

Figure 9.13. Pressure bands for assisting with pharyngoesophageal segment formation in patients having insufficient segment resistance (*hypotonicity*). (A) Elastic band with adjustable Velcro™ fastening. (B) Dan Kelly pressure band made of plastic with an adjustable elastic band and assorted pressure heads. From "Improving oesophageal communication" by J. C. Shanks, in *Laryngectomy: Diagnosis to Rehabilitation* (p. 173) by Y. Edels (Ed.), 1983, Rockville, MD: Aspen. Copyright 1983 by Yvonne Edels. Reprinted by permission.

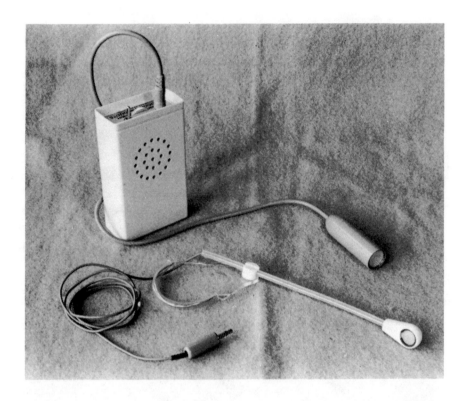

Figure 9.14. Portable speech amplifier showing both hand-held and no-hands micro-phones. From "Rehabilitation, not just voice" by G. Darvil, in *Laryngectomy: Diagnosis to Rehabilitation* (p. 201) by Y. Edels (Ed.), 1983, Rockville, MD: Aspen. Copyright 1983 by Yvonne Edels. Reprinted by permission.

fortuitous alteration in PE segment function. The literature also indicates both that the esophageal lumen can be narrowed and esophageal spasms increased by negative emotions (fear, anxiety, apprehension, and grief), and that relaxation and a consequent widening of the lumen can be caused by happiness, elation, enthusiasm, and contentment (Faulkner, 1940; Greene, 1947).

Cheesman (1987) proposed that functionally inadequate reconstruction of the PE segment due, for example, to insufficient mucosal tissue or to method of suturing when closing, can impair esophageal phonation. The relationship of surgical type and extent, and of radiotherapy, to tissue elasticity and phonatory problems, remains controversial.

Inadequate coordination of respiratory movements has also been implicated as a source of failure to develop reliable esophageal voice,

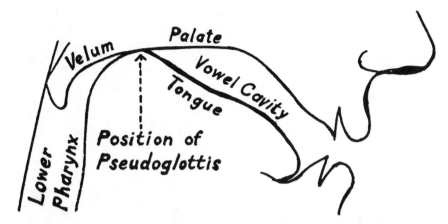

Figure 9.15. Method of producing a velar-palatal pseudoglottis. Air is collected in the lower pharynx and the tongue is raised against the velum. Air is forced out between the tongue and the velum, producing a tone. From "Speech Without Using the Larynx" by E. W. Scripture, 1916, *Journal of Physiology, 50*, p. 400. Copyright 1916 by Cambridge University Press. Reprinted by permission.

but the literature is inconclusive. Both synchrony and asynchrony reportedly occur in different and same speakers, and in injection and inhalation users, although standard injectors are more frequently synchronous. Perry (1983) stated, "Diaphragmatic problems crucially affect the acquisition of voice" (p. 182). She indicated that patients having poor respiratory movements and incoordination with neoglottic movements will not have good voices; patients with good voices tend to have coordinated movements; and varying degrees of coordination result in varying percentages of intelligible syllables.

Failure Following Esophageal Voice Acquisition. Failure after esophageal voice acquisition can also occur, notably as failure to develop esophageal speech that is readily intelligible and acceptable to the listener. Intelligible, acceptable speech is achieved primarily by refining esophageal speech skills—particularly duration, intensity, pitch, quality, articulation, and prosody—once a reliable tone is established.

Many of the physical problems described earlier can be mild enough to permit establishment of minimal esophageal phonation, but detrimental enough to preclude either vocal refinement or satisfactory articulation. These problems include strictures and pouches, PE segment hyper- or hypotonicity, labial and lingual paresis, and sensory problems, notably hearing loss. The signs, diagnosis, and management of the dis-

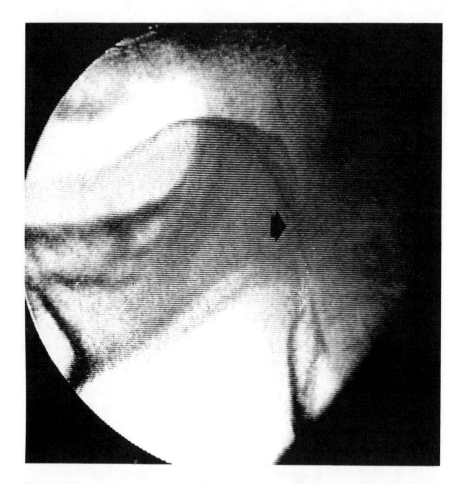

Figure 9.16. Vocal tract narrowing between the base of the tongue and the posterior pharyngeal wall (arrow) during production of pharyngeal voice in a patient (S.B.) without an adequate pharyngoesophageal segment. From "Radiographic and manometric assessment of the patient who fails to acquire esophageal voice" by E. D. Blom, in *Laryngectomee Rehabilitation* (p. 192) by R. L. Keith and F. L. Darley (Eds.), 1979, Austin, TX: PRO-ED. Copyright 1979 by PRO-ED, Inc. Reprinted by permission of PRO-ED, Inc.

orders described in Table 9.1 under problems with trapping esophageal air or producing esophageal tone, are equally applicable when they impede phonatory and articulatory refinement.

Recurring cancer is an additional source of postacquisition failure requiring clinician concern. An early sign of metastasis, which frequently occurs in the esophagus, can be sudden regression in speech, particularly reduced phonatory duration. Moreover, some evidence indicates that individuals who have had cancer are in greater jeopardy of developing other cancers. In either case, it behooves the clinician to encourage clients to see their physicians when suspicious signs occur.

Finally, failure can also occur after esophageal speech is established. To be functional, the speaker must feel reasonably competent and accepting of the changed way of speaking, as witnessed by spontaneity and consistency of oral exchange. Both the speech clinician and the client should recognize that speech-enhancing devices often can assure communication in situations limited by speaker and situational restrictions, such as excessive background noise, listener hearing loss, early stages of speech acquisition, and speaker fatigue. The speech clinician must also be aware of any social, occupational, and psychological variables impeding speech use, and direct the management program toward their eradication or reduction (Gilmore, 1986).

Social Factors

Physical disabilities can create profound changes in social relationships, including relationships with spouse and family, friends and associates, and the community. Athelstan (1981) stated that change in social status is one of the most predictable effects of a visible disability, with the disabled individual assuming a special kind of minority status, a socially devalued role, and often being presumed to be less attractive, desirable, and capable in ways that may be totally unrelated to the disability. Moreover, economic consequences of disability—for example, reduced income and depletion of family assets to pay medical expenses—can also reduce social status.

Clearly, laryngectomized individuals can be classified as disabled, often visibly, and certainly audibly. Consequently, they may be subject to significant reductions in income, social status, and satisfying interaction with family, friends, and others. Visible stigmata exist in the form of the stoma and its associated changes in breathing, coughing, and eliminating mucus; changes following radical neck dissection in neck size and configuration, or in shoulder elevation and range of arm movement; and facial grimaces, visible air-trapping maneuvers, or digital manipulation of the neck, associated with speech production. Audibly, the laryngectomized speaker demonstrates spectral and temporal speech changes reflecting modifications in the air supply, vibratory source, and resonatory tract. Noises associated with air trapping (clicks and klunks) and egress of air from the stoma can distract and disturb the listener, as well as mask speech that may already be suffering from reduced intensity. Indeed, the laryngectomized individual's differences "become patent when he is asked to speak, cough, breathe, eat, smell, bathe, lift, cry, or laugh" (Diedrich & Youngstrom, 1966, p. 66).

Family Relationships. Spouse and family relationships can facilitate speech through patience, support, understanding, reinforcement, and motivation during numerous adjustments that must be accomplished by the laryngectomized individual. This support is especially important during initial speech attempts, and while speech is being refined. Conversely, a number of potentially interrelated spouse and family problems, some predating and others originating or exacerbating with laryngectomy, can hinder speech rehabilitation.

Alterations in lifestyle related to health, occupation, finances, social contacts, and family roles and dynamics, can be primary trouble sources. Because of the laryngectomy, fathers may be forced to relinquish breadwinner roles to mothers, who, in assuming those roles, must relegate caretaker responsibilities to children. Children may feel burdened by responsibilities their peers do not have, and cheated of the maternal indulgence and economic advantages their peers enjoy. Fathers may feel guilty, see themselves as failures in "the male role," and feel frustrated in assuming roles "normally expected of the mother." Sexual problems can aggravate, or be aggravated by, these changes.

Difficulties also may be attributable to attitudes and behaviors of both the laryngectomized person and family members, including problems reflecting poor speech intelligibility, rejection of new speech modes (esophageal or mechanical–electrical), and embarrassment, as well as maladjustments consequent to inadequate preparation and counseling. These problems are reflected, for instance, in concerns expressed by laryngectomized women regarding their husbands' avoidance of them, excessive pity, and "babying" responses (Gardner, 1966). All of these can undermine progress toward functional speech through family frustration, resentment, and overprotectiveness, and through laryngectomee depression, inaccessibility, withdrawal, or dependency.

Other Social Relationships. Relationships with friends and associates following laryngectomy are subject to the same social adjustment changes described by Cogswell (1967) regarding a group of spinal cord injured men: dissolution of previous friendships, and marked reductions in frequency of entering community settings, number of roles played, and social contacts. In brief, social relationships can be characterized by withdrawal.

Nicholson (1975), a laryngectomized writer, epitomized the dynamics of withdrawal as she described her sensitivity, embarrassment, and defensiveness. She recounted her struggle to retain her sense of humor, and to accept both herself and the unknowing, inquisitive, and frequently intended-to-help behaviors of others.

The literature corroborates clinical reports of perceived family and friend discomfort in the presence of the laryngectomized individual, and of the individual's own embarrassment, avoidance of speaking to prevent notice by others, and self-imposed isolation to prevent exposure to rejection. Even trusted friends may be shunned when they have hearing losses that make an already difficult communication task more difficult; when one's bids at bridge are slow or difficult to decode; when the friendship has revolved around strenuous sports, especially water sports; or when friendly meals together require simultaneous eating and speaking.

Interest and participation in church, civic, political, and community service activities are often reduced following laryngectomy, and passive involvements increased. Those who live alone (e.g., the elderly widowed) may have both little need to speak and little opportunity to practice. One notable exception, participation in laryngectomee support groups and the International Association of Laryngectomees, may counter the lack of interests and hobbies and the isolation reported by clients and researchers.

Community Status. Problems of social stigma and rejection are encountered in the community as well as in the home and the friendly gathering. Reports by clients are validated by studies indicating that laryngectomized individuals are often relegated to inferior status. Speech pathologists, social workers, and rehabilitation counselors have demonstrated inadequate knowledge and experience, and consequent attitudes that impede social acceptance and rehabilitation (Killarney & Lass, 1979). Esophageal speakers have been perceived as being able to hold fewer positions, and primarily ones entailing less social contact and less prestige than matched laryngeal speakers, and they also were relegated to more distant social relationships (Gilmore, 1974).

In summary, being laryngectomized can have extensive social repercussions that involve the spouse, family, friends, and general community. Since both the needs and the rewards for communication derive from social interaction, its impairment can impede speech development. Withdrawal *precludes* a need for speech, as well as opportunities to practice and generalize new skills, experience success, and develop confidence.

Occupational Factors

Vocational and avocational activities constitute the major ways in which time is occupied. Occupation relates to speech acquisition in ways that parallel the relationship between social factors and speech acquisition, notably as a generator of need to speak, opportunity to practice, and reward for progress. Client reports and the literature indicate that occupational changes resulting from laryngectomy are another potential source of problems that restrict speech acquisition.

Changes in Employment. Employment changes, including retirement, job loss, demotion, or transfer, frequently follow loss of the larynx. Discrimination has often been reported as a reason for failure to retain an old position or to find a new one. Reduced public contact and job responsibility, especially in supervision of others, can reflect either employer misconceptions regarding disabilities or insidious overprotection of an "old and deserving" worker. Early retirement or job loss can also arouse doubts about one's value or worthiness, especially if one subscribes to the work ethic. Reductions in income, recognition, status, satisfaction, and self-esteem often accompany reductions in opportunities to speak and to develop confidence. All potentially heighten grief and compromise motivation.

Employment is acknowledged not only as a prime source of motivation to speak, but also as a potential determinant of the mode of speech to be developed. Individuals are often encountered who opt to develop artificial larynx or tracheoesophageal speech because these modes potentially require less time to become functional, and consequently shorten the time before return to work is possible. In this sense, motivation to return to work rapidly may preclude acquiring esophageal speech.

Avocational Activities. Like vocational pursuits, avocational interests and activities can be curtailed by physical changes. Old hobbies can be precluded by inability to work around sawdust or spray paints because of the stoma. Sports may no longer be pursued because of reduced endurance or concern for proximity to water. Restrictions in intelligibility while speech is being learned, in vocal intensity, and in simultaneously dining and conversing, can increase feelings of frustration, failure, and withdrawal from group recreational activities. Avocational reduction is reported by clients and in the literature, and with it reductions in speech needs and opportunities, and personal satisfaction.

Psychological Factors

The sudden and extensive physical, social, and occupational changes associated with laryngectomy can precipitate a series of identity crises and generate considerable stress as the individual and the family struggle to cope and to adjust to them. The resulting emotions, attitudes, and behaviors can be significant both as sources or as results of speech failure. They also can be effectively managed in programs where they are anticipated and recognized. Few laryngectomized patients need psychiatric referral.

Emotion and Motivation. Psychological factors affecting speech acquisition can be classified as emotional or motivational (Gardner, 1971). Terms used to connote motivation include effort, energy, willingness to work, industry, willingness to learn, self-discipline, fortitude, and determination. Motivation is a universally recognized prerequisite for learning and behavior change. It has been acknowledged as indispensible for mastering esophageal speech, and as the primary determinant of speech intelligibility. Clients lacking motivation are presumed to be unable to accomplish the extent and duration of effort and cooperation required for speech rehabilitation.

Premorbid psychosocial status—the individual's social and psychological traits prior to laryngectomy—can be significant determinants of postsurgical emotional factors. Sako, Cardinale, Marchetta, and Shedd (1974) suggested that the psychological concomitants of laryngectomy can be viewed as the magnification of presurgical emotional problems by the trauma and stress associated with laryngeal cancer.

Socioeconomic status can have disparate effects. Elevated educational, vocational, and social standing can reflect intellect, sophistication, and interpersonal skills that either promote rehabilitation or portend traumatic loss of status that impedes it. Modest educational background can either reduce adaptive resources, or increase motivation to regain speech because reading and writing levels preclude them as communication options. In short, socioeconomic variables are influential, but can operate in an "either–or" fashion. Their dynamics should be assessed independently for each client.

Presurgical psychological traits of significance for speech rehabilitation include introversion, inhibition, rigidity, dependence, lack of persistence, patterns of maladjustment (alcohol abuse, inability to support the family, poor relations with neighbors, anxiety, etc.), and lack of motivation. Moreover, preexistent psychological traits can be magnified by the new situation and its associated trauma, resulting in significant emotional problems.

Critical Phases. Several writers have attempted to substantiate clinical impressions that emotional reactions following laryngectomy reflect temporal, crisis-associated phases of readjustment (Gardner, 1966; Locke, 1966; Sanchez-Salazar & Stark, 1972). Clinicians generally agree that the initial crisis involves reactions to the diagnosis of cancer and the disease itself. The psychological impact of having cancer, particularly laryngeal cancer, can be overwhelming. Some reject the alaryngeal voice and the surgery. Fear, apprehension, and anxiety regarding loss are likely to be dominant early responses. The anticipated loss of voice, job, friends, family, status, and potentially even life itself, can seem insurmountable. The responses attending diagnosis of cancer can include passive resignation, self-pity, ego deflation, anxiety, insomnia, irritability, seclusiveness, confusion, depression, withdrawal, and suicidal tendencies.

The second crucial phase occurs after surgery, when the individual realizes and appreciates the changes and restrictions imposed by the surgery, notably the loss of speech. Laryngectomized clients frequently and vividly recall their initial and probably most traumatic experience of this phase: waking up in the recovery room aware of the equipment designed to maintain respiration, and being unable to call for help. Death remains a significant fear, as well as fears of cancer recurrence, old age, and uselessness due to speech loss. Depression and feelings of desolation are often expressed, and increased dependency and withdrawal are not infrequent during this phase.

Later crises include (a) occasions entailing reductions in protection and attentiveness (e.g., when leaving the hospital or when convalescence is completed); (b) occasions calling for initial public appearances and consequent acknowledgment of the physical, social, and psychological concomitants of being a laryngectomee; and (c) occasions during rehabilitation and readjustment that evoke emotional reactions (e.g., confronting required use of an artificial larynx, or vocational and avocational changes necessitated by having a stoma). The third stage could be viewed as a rehabilitation phase, when crises reflect the fears, conflicts, frustrations, and compromises associated with gaining independence and coming to terms with one's status. The emotional responses characterizing this phase are sensitivity, feeling disfigured, anxiety, embarrassment, depression, and perhaps seclusiveness and withdrawal. Reductions in motivation, real or apparent, can accompany these emotions.

If rehabilitation is perceived to be in jeopardy, the associated reactions can include heightened resentment of the physical changes, especially the stoma; loss of self-esteem; feelings of inferiority and rejection; loss of interest in the world and self; and perhaps abandonment of speech efforts. Fears of loss of job, money, friends, and prestige may be aggravated. Depression may deepen as it reflects social and economic barriers and burdens imposed by the lack of speech.

Perhaps the temporal nature of the reactions and adjustments following loss of the larynx is best described in the grieving process model. Shontz (1965) proposed a model involving a series of five stages or phrases of adjustment, each accompanied by a characteristic emotional experience. The predominant emotional reaction changes as the individual progresses through the five stages: shock, realization, defensive retreat, acknowledgment, and adaptation.

Nicholson (1975) described her own reactions to her pre- and postoperative experiences during her first 2 years. Prior to surgery she felt shock and numbness, loss related to trading her voice for a "makeshift," fear of surgery, repulsion for the disfigurement, and gratefulness for family support. Following the surgery she felt the "relentless impact of voicelessness" as though she was "imprisoned by silence," defeat due to failing to develop satisfactory esophageal speech, a "love–hate relationship" with her artificial larynx, and annoyance and embarrassment with her inability to sing, laugh aloud, smell, swim, suck soup from a spoon, blow out birthday candles, and call out for help in danger. She described her most grievous losses as a "forfeiture of personality," which she attributed to communicating so poorly, being "bereft . . . of repartee with others," and "infrequent cruelties, such as when strangers hang up on the phone or laugh thinking it's a joke." She indicated that there were still times of depression, but that they were decreasing as time went by. She concluded, "I shall adjust to the brokenness and deprivations inherent in my present status" (p. 2158).

Understanding the critical stages confronting the laryngectomized individual can do much more to reduce speech failure. Most obviously, a preventive approach can be structured and staffed to deal with anticipated patient and family reactions. For instance, direct speech training may be minimized during early stages, and efforts directed primarily at providing ventilation, support, and answering questions.

Increased clinician sensitivity to anticipated client reactions can minimize problems that might otherwise reduce the energy available for speech therapy, or undermine the motivation to drill, practice, or pursue speech at all. It has often been observed that time spent in ventilating feelings can actually shorten time-to-task. Letting bad feelings out *can* help good feelings sprout, as well as generate new adaptive strategies.

Awareness of crucial phases can have another clinical value: "normalization" of behavior. Emotional reactions following laryngectomy are likely to be reactive and temporary rather than characteristic personality patterns. They often can be dealt with through ventilation, support, and helping the individual and the family to devise strategies for coping. Otherwise, as the literature too frequently indicates, failing clients are written off as helpless, dependent, unwilling to assume responsibility for their own care, lacking motivation and drive, and as passive personalities whose sense of well-being depends on cigarettes or alcohol.

Training Factors

The last category of problems contributing to failure, training factors, has two divisions: problems of clinician competence and problems of program comprehensiveness. Both reflect the complexity and the uniqueness of the array of variables affecting postlaryngectomy rehabilitation. In short, postlaryngectomy speech rehabilitation is sufficiently unlike managing any other single communication disorder in which specialized study, experience, and management resources are required.

Postlaryngectomy speech changes reflect the fact that respiration, phonation, articulation, and resonance are all affected. Vocal duration and intensity, speech rate, and prosodic variation are all constrained. The competent speech clinician must have knowledge and skills regarding all of these speech parameters and their relationship to esophageal voice, and to esophageal speech once voice is established. Additionally, knowledge and appreciation of the psychosocial and physical factors impeding speech acquisition are required to the extent that the dynamics can be assessed and a program devised to eliminate, minimize, or compensate for them.

Program comprehensiveness is demanded by the complexity of the postlaryngectomy rehabilitation task. An array of disciplines is required to manage the variety of psychosocial and physical problems discussed previously. Moreover, to be most effective, each discipline requires significant knowledge regarding the functions and procedures of the others to be able to provide information, opportunities for ventilation, support, reinforcement, and direction to laryngectomized patients and their families.

Idiopathic Factors

Idiopathic is a medical term indicating that a given disorder is thought to be self-originated, or to have occurred without known cause. Duguay (1986) has used OGK—Only God Knows—to refer to those few individuals for whom specific reasons for failure to acquire speech cannot be ascertained. Idiopathic factors are acknowledged in this section for two reasons. The first is to indicate that although extensive, the list of factors discussed in the chapter is neither all-inclusive nor *routinely* applicable. The second is to comfort the clinician faced with a difficult client. There is still much to be learned clinically and through research.

SUMMARY AND CONCLUSIONS

Unresolved and perplexing questions remain regarding why approximately 40% of laryngectomized individuals fail to develop esophageal speech, and what distinguishes them from the successful speakers and from the 15% who are superior. Two schools of thought exist: those who see the problems as being primarily physical, and those who feel that psychological factors underlie success or failure.

The physical school is focused on the capability of the residual vocal tract to support effective speech. Consequently, these clinicians are concerned with the effects of such factors as type and extent of medical treatment; posttreatment morbidity; and pre- or postsurgical structural and physiological problems related to trapping air, phonating, and refining speech. The psychological school is concerned with psychosocial alterations and adjustments. These clinicians argue that the inability either to establish physical reasons for speech failure in some clients, or to explain why others speak well despite extensive surgery or postoperative complications, demonstrates the significance of psychosocial factors in speech success and failure.

A third group of factors contributing to failure, inadequate training, includes both program comprehensiveness and clinician competence. Doubtless, both physical and psychosocial factors contribute to failure, often in the same individual. The crucial question is whether they are anticipated or discovered before they result in frustration, loss of motivation, withdrawal, and failure.

A successful speech rehabilitation program involves the array of disciplines and competencies necessary to manage the variety of factors that can impede postlaryngectomy rehabilitation. Moreover, it is preventively oriented, which is demonstrated in two ways. With regard to physical problems, preventive approaches provide either pretherapy probes or early assessment when difficulties are encountered, to ensure that the residual vocal tract is capable of supporting esophageal speech. These procedures include X-ray evaluation and air insufflation testing, in particular. When indicated, medical remediation is provided early. With regard to psychosocial factors, preventive approaches routinely include educational, counseling, and support programs, especially during the initial stages of adjustment and management. Additionally, probing and assessment procedures are employed to uncover patterns of maladjustment or other psychosocial problems, and treatment is instituted before patterns of speech failure become firmly entrenched.

Finally, it should be recognized that many of the factors impeding esophageal speech acquisition are potent causes of failure to acquire *any form* of alaryngeal speech, be it by means of an artificial larynx or a tracheoesophageal puncture. Competent staff and comprehensive programs help to assure success and prevent failure regardless of speech mode.

REFERENCES

Athelstan, G. (1981). Psychosocial adjustment to chronic disease and disability. In W. Stolov & M. Flowers (Eds.), *Handbook of severe disability* (pp. 13–18). Washington, DC: U.S. Department of Education, Rehabilitation Services Administration.

Blom, E. D. (1979). Radiographic and manometric assessment of the patient who fails to acquire esophageal voice. In R. L. Keith & F. L. Darley (Eds.), *Laryngectomee rehabilitation* (pp. 181–204). Austin, TX: PRO-ED.

Cheesman, A. D. (1987, August). *Case presentation and surgical procedure.* Paper presented at the First National Laryngectomee Rehabilitation Seminar, Melbourne, Australia.

Cogswell, B. (1967). Rehabilitation of the paraplegic: Processes of socialization. *Sociology Inquiry, 37,* 11–26.

Darvill, G. (1983). Rehabilitation—Not just voice. In Y. Edels (Ed.), *Laryngectomy: Diagnosis to rehabilitation* (pp. 192–217). Rockville, MD: Aspen.

Diedrich, W., & Youngstrom, K. (1966). *Alaryngeal speech.* Springfield, IL: Charles C. Thomas.

Duguay, M. (1986). Special problems of the alaryngeal speaker. In R. L. Keith & F. L. Darley (Eds.), *Laryngectomee rehabilitation* (2nd. ed., pp. 309–321). Austin, TX: PRO-ED.

Faulkner, W. B. (1940). Objective esophageal changes due to psychic factors. *American Journal of Medical Sciences, 200,* 796–803.

Finkbeiner, E. R. (1974). Surgery and speech, the pseudoglottis, and respiration in total standard laryngectomy. In J. C. Snidecor (Ed.), *Speech rehabilitation of the laryngectomized* (2nd ed., pp. 58–85). Springfield, IL: Charles C. Thomas.

Fox, D. D. (1986). Clinical considerations in management of the laryngectomee. In R. L. Keith & F. L. Darley (Eds.), *Laryngectomee rehabilitation* (2nd ed., pp. 371–400). Austin, TX: PRO-ED.

Gardner, W. (1966). Adjustment problems of laryngectomized women. *Archives of Otolaryngology, 83,* 31–42.

Gardner, W. (1971). *Laryngectomee speech and rehabilitation.* Springfield, IL: Charles C. Thomas.

Gates, G., & Hearne, E. (1982). Predicting esophageal speech. *Annals of Otology, Rhinology and Laryngology, 91,* 454–457.

Gates, G., Ryan, W., Cantu, E., & Hearne, E. (1982). Current status of laryngectomee rehabilitation: II. Causes of failure. *American Journal of Otolaryngology, 3,* 8–14.

Gates, G., Ryan, W., Cooper, J., Lawlis, G., Cantu, E., Hayashi, T., Lauder, E., Welch, R., & Hearne, E. (1982). Current status of laryngectomee rehabilitation: I. Results of therapy. *American Journal of Otolaryngology, 3,* 1–7.

Gates, G., Ryan, W., & Lauder, E. (1982). Current status of laryngectomee rehabilitation: IV. Attitudes about laryngectomee rehabilitation should change. *American Journal of Otolaryngology, 3,* 97–103.

Gilmore, S. (1974). Social and vocational acceptability of esophageal speakers compared to normal speakers. *Journal of Speech and Hearing Research, 17,* 599–607.

Gilmore, S. (1986). The psychosocial concomitants of laryngectomy. In R. L. Keith & F. L. Darley (Eds.), *Laryngectomee rehabilitation* (2nd ed., pp. 425–495). Austin, TX: PRO-ED.

Greene, J. S. (1947). Laryngectomy and its psychologic implications. *New York State Journal of Medicine, 47,* 53–56.

Killarney, G., & Lass, N. (1979). A comparative study of the knowledge, exposure and attitude of speech pathologists, rehabilitation counselors and social workers toward laryngectomized individuals. *Journal of Rehabilitation, 44,* 34–38.

Kirchner, J. A., Scatliff, J. H., Dey, F. L., & Shedd, D. P. (1963). The pharynx after laryngectomy: Changes in its structure and function. *Laryngoscope, 73,* 18–33.

Locke, B. (1966). Psychology of the laryngectomee. *Military Medicine, 131,* 593–599.

Logemann, J. A. (1983). Extensive surgery for post-cricoid carcinoma and subsequent vocal rehabilitation: B. Vocal rehabilitation after extensive surgery for post-cricoid carcinoma. In Y. Edels (Ed.), *Laryngectomy: Diagnosis to rehabilitation* (pp. 233–248). Rockville, MD: Aspen.

McGarvey, S. D., & Weinberg, B. (1984). Esophageal insufflation testing in non-laryngectomized adults. *Journal of Speech and Hearing Disorders, 49,* 272–277.

Nicholson, E. (1975). Personal notes of a laryngectomee. *American Journal of Nursing, 75,* 2157–2158.

Perry, A. (1983). Difficulties in the acquisition of alaryngeal speech. In Y. Edels (Ed.), *Laryngectomy: Diagnosis to rehabilitation* (pp. 177–191). Rockville, MD: Aspen Publications.

Ranger, D. (1983). Extensive surgery for post-cricoid carcinoma and subsequent vocal rehabilitation: A. Extensive surgery for post-cricoid carcinoma. In Y. Edels (Ed.), *Laryngectomy: Diagnosis to rehabilitation* (pp. 218–232). Rockville, MD: Aspen.

Sako, K., Cardinale, S., Marchetta, F., & Shedd, D. (1974). Speech and vocational rehabilitation of the laryngectomized patient. *Journal of Surgical Oncology, 6,* 197–202.

Sanchez-Salazar, V., & Stark, A. (1972). The use of crisis intervention in the rehabilitation of laryngectomees. *Journal of Speech and Hearing Disorders, 37,* 323–328.

Scripture, E. W. (1916). Speech without using the larynx. *Journal of Physiology, 50,* 397–403.

Shanks, J. C. (1983). Improving oesophageal communication. In Y. Edels (Ed.), Laryngectomy: Diagnosis to rehabilitation (pp. 163–176). Rockville, MD: Aspen.

Shontz, F. (1965). Reactions of crisis. *Volta Review, 67,* 364–370.

Simpson, I., Smith, J., & Gordon, M. (1972). Laryngectomy: The influence of muscle reconstruction on the mechanism of oesophageal voice production. *Journal of Laryngology and Otology, 86,* 961–990.

Singer, M., & Blom, E. (1981). Selective myotomy for voice restoration after total laryngectomy. *Archives of Otolaryngology, 107,* 670–673.

Volin, R. (1980). Predicting failure to speak after laryngectomy. *Laryngoscope, 90,* 1727–1736.

Winans, C. S., Reichbach, E. J., & Waldrop, W. F. (1974). Esophageal determinants of alaryngeal speech. *Archives of Otolaryngology, 88,* 10–14.

CHAPTER 10

Living with a Laryngectomee

Martha Strasser

Strasser's chapter is unique because it is the only chapter written by the spouse of a laryngectomee that has been published. She presents an unusual viewpoint because she is able to speak both as a spouse and as a teacher of alaryngeal speech in Germany. Although the issues discussed are presented only from her perspective, she highlights some concerns to all spouses of laryngectomized individuals.

Study Questions

1. Should the patient or spouse expect an esophageal sound during the first therapy session?
2. Would you have the spouse attend every speech therapy session?
3. What attitudes or behaviors are important when working with laryngectomees?

More than 30 years have passed since my husband was told that he had cancer of the larynx and that in order to save his life he would have to undergo an operation called a laryngectomy. Because the voice box would be removed during this operation, he would not be able to talk anymore. I will try in recollection to give an honest answer to all the questions and problems that arose after this diagnosis was made.

By talking of "honest," I mean two different "truths." First is the story about the different changes of lifestyle my husband and all of the family had to experience, realize, and accept up to his death. Second is the difficulty of talking openly about the change of relationship that occurred after this operation.

It is the custom, and I believe a good and helpful custom, that a spouse does not complain in public about the other spouse. Yet here I am trying to put in writing what I felt and experienced after having lived for 14 years with a laryngectomee. By describing problems, changes, and difficult reactions, I hope I might help in the successful rehabilitation of other laryngectomees and their families.

CHANGES OF LIFESTYLE

In 1957 my husband was 50 years old and had been an independent representative of a well-known textile company in the state of Bavaria, Federal Republic of Germany. Together with his 30 employees he worked hard, nearly day and night, including weekends, smoked, and was successful. Early in 1957 his company decided to change the selling system. Instead of using independent representatives, the company employed directors with good pay and pension. This change did not suit my husband, who was proud of having achieved so much, since the start of German economics after World War II. He resigned and planned to find another worthwhile textile distributorship. Thus he had more time and could finally go to the otorhinolaryngologist, as he had been hoarse for many weeks, even months.

The diagnosis was cancer of the larynx with all the consequences. Being an independent man, he had gone alone to the doctor and I heard the news through him. The family—my husband, five children (ages 4, 6, 10, 19, and 20), and I—were living in an old comfortable house approximately 20 miles south of Munich. I remember this "newsbreaking" very well. We were sitting in the garden, and my husband simply said, "I have cancer; the larynx has to be removed, meaning I will not be able to talk anymore."

What did I feel? Not a fear of the word cancer. Perhaps because I was the daughter of a missionary doctor, the word cancer did not sound so dangerous. I knew very well that an operation could help. I did not immediately understand what it meant not to be able to talk anymore. So I felt relieved, because I had been concerned about my husband's health and hoarseness. I had also been previously warned by his doctor that considering the way my husband was working at the age of 50, a heart attack could occur any time. My thought was, "This operation forces you to calm down, think of your health, and also have more time for the family." Besides that, the doctor had told him the tumor was small and located on only one of the vocal cords.

The next step was a biopsy, which proved the cancer. Radiation treatment was suggested. Remember, this was 1957 and the medical–technical possibilities were not as developed as they are today. During all this time I had not met the doctor. During the 6 weeks of radiation therapy, I drove my husband to the hospital and back, but he wanted his independence and refused my company within the hospital.

After 3 months, my husband came home from a visit to the doctor and reported that the tumor had vanished and that the doctor had suggested going on a vacation to recover from the radiation. Nevertheless, my husband was asked to have a checkup every 3 weeks.

We were planning to visit France, where my husband had been stationed for many years during World War II. Being able to speak French, he had been able to communicate with the local people and liked them very much. He wanted to see all the old places again.

About 8 days before we were to leave, a phone call came. By chance I answered the phone. The head nurse who worked for my husband's doctor asked at once, "Are you alone?" When I stated I was, she asked me to visit the doctor at a certain time in the next few days, without telling my husband. Naturally I was alarmed. At the meeting I was told that at the last checkup the tumor was visible again and that the life-saving operation was absolutely necessary. The doctor apologized that he was telling me this alone, but he thought this the best way, especially as he also had wanted to meet me. He said we should go on our vacation but report to the hospital as soon as we were back.

At this point I felt shocked, stunned. With whom should I talk? Should I tell this "news" before the holiday? Many feelings, fears, and questions arose which could not be answered. At least I was able to contact at once one of my husband's good friends who was also a doctor. He tried to calm me down and said that he would call the otorhinolaryngologist to get more information, and that in the meantime I should go on holiday with my husband.

And this is what we did. I admit, I not only do not remember much about this trip to France, but I certainly could not enjoy it, knowing what was expected of us in Germany.

Back home again, my husband's operation was on November 27, 1957. I was able to stay with him day and night after the hospital staff noticed that I, with the help of the nurse, could really be of assistance. Yes, I must admit, all the different "equipment" was new to me; however, I did not mind the stoma. I got used to the coughing and the mucus, I learned to handle the suction machine, and so forth. My first positive experience was that communication still was possible. My husband whispered, and when I was close to him, alone with him in the room, I could understand him. Very soon I began to learn to lipread. The operation was "normal," as the medical people call it, only 4 hr long. Instead of being able to go home after 2 or 3 weeks as planned, however, my husband developed a fistula. A nasal feeding tube was inserted, and my husband had to stay 2 months in the hospital. Due to the preoperative radiation the healing process was disturbed, which, according to the medical staff, contributed to the development of the fistula.

Finally my husband could leave the hospital. We were both happy but nervous. We wondered about the family's reaction and about how everything would go.

Here, I believe it is time to explain why I could stay with my husband in the hospital all 8 weeks. Luckily, I had two elderly housekeepers, who had lived with my parents-in-law all their lives and who continued to work for us, living with us in the house. As mentioned earlier, my husband had been earning enough money during the years before the operation that the financial situation at that time was not a problem. Thus I was free to care for my husband. I was thankful for this time together, especially as one of the first sentences he whispered to me after the operation was, "Now I am an old disabled man; you can look for a young man!" My natural reaction was to stay with him as much as possible, to show how little my love had changed, and to prove that I was not looking for a young and healthy man. Before detailing the change in our relationship, however, let me state in a few sentences how we managed to carry on the outward life of the family.

At that time speech pathologists/logopedes were unknown in Germany. My husband could not talk for more than 3 years, but he eventually learned esophageal speech on his own, after meeting a laryngectomee who spoke this way. The two of us started several of our own businesses, ultimately representing textile again. We could then take advantage of my husband's old business connections. Together, we earned enough money to raise the three young children, give them the necessary education, keep the house, and stay independent. After several years, however, my husband developed heart insufficiency which, although treated, did not improve. Due to this weakness, I believe, he

one day fell and broke his upper leg; although his bone was successfully nailed in the hospital, he passed away in early January 1971.

CHANGES OF RELATIONSHIP

The most stringent change is a laryngectomee's inability to talk with
voice anymore, but also a stoma is difficult to accept. As mentioned
earlier, I did not mind these changes at all. Certainly, one has to get
used to the mucus that comes from coughing directly out of the stoma.
The laryngectomee has to learn to keep a tissue at hand to wipe away
this mucus. Even better, the person can wear a stomacover, which should
fit well and be kept clean. It is very hard for the laryngectomee to hold
back his or her coughing. The trachea also has to be kept clean so that
air can pass freely into the lungs. When leaving the hospital, most
patients still need a tracheostomy tube, which also should be kept clean.
Certainly, the importance of hygiene has to be explained to the patient
and spouse in the hospital, but the laryngectomee is responsible from
the start for appearance. A small mirror and a handkerchief to keep
together in a pocket make a nice present and help when the patient
leaves the hospital.

Breathing and coughing both sound different following a laryngectomy, but this should not cause fear when a bedcovering slips over the
stoma. Many people sleep with their heads, and consequently their noses,
covered, and they do not suffocate. The stoma is the new, "artificial"
nose for a laryngectomee. Therefore, it is not true when laryngectomees
state that they do not get enough air when using a stomacover. Certainly, they need good stomacovers, which not only help laryngectomees
look clean and tidy, but also filter the inhaled air and add the necessary moisture to the breath.

The most difficult thing for me was to always have my husband at
home, watching every step I took and always expecting me to be available and ready to help if necessary. It is a very natural reaction for the
patient at home to feel lost. Everyday life changes for the laryngectomee,
the spouse, and the family. Laryngectomees often feel helpless. Not only
do they not want to admit this helpless feeling, but such feelings often
are contrary to their way of life before the operation. The laryngectomee's inability to verbalize wishes or talk about feelings causes irri-
tations, impatience, aggressiveness, or withdrawal. Naturally, these
problems disturb the whole family pattern.

My husband did not want to see or talk to anyone. He instructed
me to ask his friends, both personal and business, not to come either
to the hospital or, later, to our home. Not knowing better, I accepted

this. Please remember that from his first words after the operation, I heard and felt his jealousy. Also, as a loving, inexperienced spouse, I accepted all his wishes. Perhaps the age difference (my husband was 14 years older) was one reason. Additionally, I believe that most laryngectomees lose a lot of their self-confidence, and it takes time to regain it.

I have to admit that my husband was never again like the man I married, loved, and tried hard to show I still loved, even though he learned to talk again after a few years and was able to earn money again. His own question, "Can you still love me and have sexual intercourse despite this terrible hole?" showed me how lost he felt. Naturally, I proved at the next possible moment by having sexual intercourse with him that my love had not changed. As the years went on, however— remember he passed away 14 years after the operation—he grew more and more depressed, showed resignation, and even said he should have refused the operation.

Was this a total change of character? Was it due to the heart problems? I do not know. I tried to encourage him by saying, "You can talk again; you or we together can earn money again; you have five healthy children; we can keep our house and do not have too many financial problems. Can't you see these positives and be thankful?" His answer was, "I would give all these things away, if in return I could have my old voice back again." And when I asked, "Even the children and I are not worth it?" his answer was "No, if all this I could achieve again!" This reply naturally hurt; it was such a blow, I could not respond.

As time passed he lost more and more interest in life. Certainly the additional heart trouble was one reason for his resignation. I could not let him drive the car alone; a certain diet had to be kept; he could drink no more than 2 liters of fluid a day. All this made him feel more helpless, and my reaction was not always the right one. Especially the last 3 to 4 years before he passed away, I was asked not only to be a loving wife, but also a trained nurse (e.g., giving shots when needed). Also, I was expected to be an independent businesswoman, earning the living and trying to keep the agency running. Additionally, two of our five children were still at home and attending the local high school.

To complete the family picture, I should mention the reaction of the children. Yes, I do think being suddenly confronted with a sick father, who not only has a "hole" in his neck, but can hardly communicate, does affect the children. Depending on the age and personality of each child, the experience and reaction vary.

During the most difficult time, approximately 3 to 4 years before my husband passed away, the three oldest children, my stepchildren, had left home and were taking care of themselves. Also, my oldest son was close to becoming a medical doctor. Only our two youngest daughters were still at home. They must have felt very peculiar when I had to ask them to stay away from school to take care of their father. The headmaster of the high school accepted my "excuses," after I explained to him the necessity. My husband in the last years could hardly be left alone at home longer than 1 or 2 hr. Not only because of his physical health, but because he became more and more sclerotic, his memory diminished. Occasionally I had to leave the house for a day to earn money and leave him with the children. My husband's state of mind was hard not only for me, but for the children as well.

Our son, the medical student, was living in Munich and working hard to finish as soon as possible. Although my two youngest daughters, who were between the ages of 14 and 18 years, helped me when I asked them and never complained, they must have suffered severely watching their father growing older and more helpless with every day. Even now, 19 years after their father passed away, when the oldest daughter, who lives in a house next to mine with her husband and two young sons, invites me to her place for a party with friends, she loves to make the remark, "Remember I am glad to have you, but please, do not mention once the word laryngectomee." And the youngest daughter, being very sensitive and mentally not as stable as the other children, likes to say, "Oh, your only interest is the 'Larry's.' I don't want to hear them talk or listen to you talking about them."

I have not yet mentioned one very important and helpful factor to both my husband and me: successful establishment of the Munich Laryngectomee Club in 1968. In the spring of 1968 we had the opportunity to visit the so-called First European Laryngectomee Meeting in Strasbourg, France. This meeting was organized mainly by French and Italian laryngectomees. My husband was very much impressed and inspired when we, together with our two youngest daughters, returned home. Approximately 200 laryngectomees attended. Some presentations were made by laryngectomees and some by medical or paramedical staff. On the 4-hr drive home, my husband said, "This is the first time since the operation that I felt at home, at ease! Why don't we have something like this in Germany?"

At the next checkup with the otorhinolaryngologist, my husband reported about this Strasbourg meeting and asked if we could have the names of other laryngectomees to at least get to know each other. Dr. Kressner agreed and congratulated my husband on his good esophageal speech. He added, "Didn't I tell you that you would learn it? All you needed was endurance and patience to have this success!" After the operation, I accompanied my husband to all the checkups. When I heard the doctor's statement, I contradicted him. I said, "It was not endurance and patience alone that helped my husband to talk. If he had not met the other laryngectomees in France who were intelligible esophageal speakers, he would not have had this success. Even if you, Dr. Kressner, tell your patient, 'You can talk again,' this does not help much. The patient needs proof by hearing another laryngectomee." I then asked, "May we come regularly and visit your laryngectomy patients and let my husband talk to them?" Dr. Kressner agreed, and this was the start not only of founding the Munich Laryngectomee Club, but also of hospital visitations, and of having a medical doctor as club president in 1968. For tax-exemption purposes, it was necessary to have a doctor as president. My husband and I invited the first 15 laryngectomees in October 1968, and they came and all agreed to be members and to register the club.

Visiting recently laryngectomized patients in the hospital always helped my husband when he felt depressed. I could always say to him, "Let's visit the hospital. I am certain you can help and encourage a patient who is just going through this bad experience." When we arrived at the hospital for our visits, we reported to the nurse or doctor on duty. This hospital, being a well-known center for head and neck patients, nearly always had a new laryngectomee. Many of them did not believe that my husband had lost his larynx. His appearance was normal since he always wore the Mutivoix, a French stomacover, after seeing it in Strasbourg. His speech was so good that he had to lift his cover to prove that he also had a stoma and had undergone the same operation.

I still remember a very dramatic scene of one of our visits. A blind laryngectomee was lying in his bed when my husband walked up to him and talked to him. The man started crying and whispered, "Thank you for coming. Thank you so much. This makes me believe that I can also learn to talk, carry on my work, and stay alive! I was just told that I still needed radiation. This news, together with not being able to talk, depressed me very much!" This meeting was in the afternoon, and later at home in the evening, his spouse called us and thanked us, especially my husband, for visiting. This couple lived 100 miles south of Munich, and the blind laryngectomee (a World War II veteran) had just started a practice as a physical therapist!

Why am I telling all this in detail, especially about the setting up of the laryngectomee club? Well, in 1971, my husband passed away (remember, not of cancer). At the following club meeting, to which I as secretary had invited the 35 members of record, I reported my husband's death. I wanted to hand the papers over to the next vice president or secretary. But the attending members asked me to carry on the work that I had started with my husband because I then knew more than anyone else! I accepted. That is why I am telling you all this. I have devoted the past 17 years to setting up and organizing a better rehabilitation program for laryngectomees and their families in Germany. This gives me the courage to add some suggestions and advice in the following section.

ADVICE AND SUGGESTIONS TO THE SPEECH PATHOLOGIST

I can imagine that you will be quite nervous when you are told, "Take over the next therapy. Your patient will be a newly operated laryngectomee!" But if you follow three important steps, I am certain that both the patient and you can look forward to successful speech therapy.

Although I cannot give you a "recipe," three points are very important. First, have enough time available and give your patient the feeling that you look on him or her as a human being, not only as a case, and that your concern is not the "new voice" alone. Second, watch the patient's facial and neck area very closely as he or she whispers answers to your questions about personal dates surrounding the surgery. Try to lipread. Watch the muscles moving to see how the articulation is handled. Third, not only watch, but listen between the whispering for an esophageal sound to be produced accidentally. Remember, you will be the first person who really takes the time to listen to the laryngectomee's concerns, questions, and uncertainties. Although the doctor should have explained what really was done through a laryngectomy, the patient probably did not comprehend much of what was said because many other questions were bothering him or her.

Have a set of slides or pictures at hand to show and explain in lay terms what actually has changed in the neck area. After having taught around 1,000 laryngectomees, I have found this explanation most important. I have often used the pictures in the book *Looking Forward* by Keith, Shane, Coates, and Devine (1984). Certainly, other books or pictures also show the change in the throat area after this operation. Of course, let the patient ask questions, but have him or her talk slowly and articulate well. Explain exactly what you mean by the term *articulation*. Show the lip movements by exaggerating the primary vowels. As a speech pathologist, you might have pictures or drawings of the features of the lips for the vowels. It is also very important to have a mirror at hand. The patient should see what he or she is doing right or wrong.

I like to explain in simple, everyday wording what the patient can do. Try to help the laryngectomee understand that it is important to learn as much as possible about esophageal voice production. If I am talking with a male, I very often say, "This esophageal voice or sound (not speech) we are talking of and we want to achieve comes from a small little valve that exists in your throat." Without going into details, I explain that his esophagus has a negative pressure, which is closed in at the top and the bottom by a ring of muscles. I state that science found this pressure difference to be of great importance in achieving esophageal sound, because in the mouth cavity, on top of this closed esophagus, is positive atmospheric pressure. If the patient can learn to release the negative air pressure from the esophagus toward the positive pressure in the throat and mouth, not only can this be felt but a sound can be heard, like the air coming out of the valve of a tire when opened. Men understand this usually very well. When talking to a female laryngectomee, I refer to the steam or pressure cooker. This air escaping from the esophagus is able to set the above tissue vibrating, making a sound, which then can be articulated and formed into words and speech. Remember, you can explain all this with good pictures, and at this point state again the importance of good articulation, simply with lips moving and no "sound" (stoma noise) from the lungs.

Perhaps your patient is not interested in speech yet; take your time and answer as well as possible all the questions and concerns. The patient might want to know about his or her pension and indemnity as a disabled person. Pick up the phone and try to contact the responsible office. Refer the patient to other agencies that might help, such as the International Association of Laryngectomees and the American Cancer Society. Describe stomacovers and how important they are, not only for a well-groomed look, but also for filtering and moistening the air before it reaches the lungs. Certainly, tell about the availability of an artificial larynx, if the patient has not been furnished with one already. Can you and others understand him or her with the speech device? If not, help with the placement of the device and explain the importance of developing good resonance. Again, stress that good articulation is very important. Certainly at this early stage, introducing the patient to an intelligible and well-rehabilitated laryngectomee might encourage him or her to begin esophageal speech training.

If all these points are of no interest to the laryngectomee, however, and if you notice more nervousness than interest in speech, try breathing and/or relaxation exercises. If the spouse is not visiting at the same time, ask him or her to come along the next time. The spouse might be able to give more information about what really concerns the patient.

Perhaps you will find out at the first session that your patient is thinking more of having to die soon than of being cured. You might not feel capable of talking with your patient about death and dying. But a well-rehabilitated laryngectomee, perhaps 5 to 10 years postoperative, could certainly help. I believe that many people do not think about death nowadays. With all the technical and scientific advances, we tend to feel that this science and knowledge will help us live long lives. Although we read daily in the newspaper or hear on television about car accidents and automotive technical failures, most people drive a car without thinking about the possibility of accidents for themselves.

What is the sense of life? Is it big money? Is it a career? Why did you, as a speech pathologist, decide to get this education and do this work? I am certain that you want to help people. You might prefer working with children; however, you will not only find more and more younger laryngectomees, but you will find the same rewarding feeling if you are able to help give back joy of life to a 60-, 70-, or 80-year-old laryngectomee. He or she might be your father, grandmother, or a good friend of your family. We, as human beings, all need each other, a baby as well as an adult having a "normal" life. Much more assistance is needed by the older and laryngectomized people!

Perhaps the concept of life as a rainbow might help you and the patient think about death and dying. Imagine a baby starting with all the colors on one horizon, then becoming an adult in the zenith, and returning back to earth at the end of life, much as the rainbow touches the opposite horizon. Again, however, if you do not feel like talking with the patient about death, refer him or her to a psychologist for help, or perhaps to a minister or priest.

In working with laryngectomees, you have to learn and accept early that you will be confronted with dying patients. Visit them for as long as you can. Just drop in, say a few words, and hold their hands to show that you have not forgotten them. These are only a few suggestions and remarks I would like to add to my life story.

I would like to close with a remarkable sentence I heard from an 82-year-old laryngectomized lady some years ago. I was organizing my second Munich Voice Institute, looking for patients to attend. At one of the Munich Laryngectomee Club meetings was a nice woman who had been a laryngectomee for 12 years and was beginning to have difficulty hearing and seeing, but nevertheless was talking fairly well with an electrolarynx. She stood in front of me and said, " I want to attend this voice institute. I think I have to tell you an important thing you have forgotten, Mrs. Strasser. I know I can hardly hear." (She pointed to her ears.) "My eyes are getting weaker and weaker; I cannot talk very well." (She pointed to her stoma.) "But I was not operated up in there," she said, pointing to her head, meaning her brain. She attended the voice institute. She also has been swimming with the LARKEL (LARyngectomee snorKEL) for many years.

Remember this story because it will always help a newly operated laryngectomee when he or she feels dumb and helpless. Tell the story and convince the patient that he or she has not lost intelligence or knowledge. Yes, the patient has a stoma and can hardly communicate, but he or she is still able to use the brain just as before the operation.

REFERENCE

Keith, R. L., Shane, H. C., Coates, H. L. C., & Devine, K. D. (1984). *Looking forward.* New York: Thieme-Stratton.

CHAPTER 11

Consequences of Total Laryngectomy in Daily Living Activities

James C. Shanks

Shanks's chapter underscores the amazing flexibility of the human being and the compensation of which one is capable. He explains how total laryngectomy affects nine bodily functions and describes laryngectomized individuals who have developed their own ways of compensating. Clinicians will discover many helpful suggestions for new laryngectomees as well as for those who experienced surgery many years ago.

Study Questions

1. *Surgical removal of the larynx affects each of the following* except:
   a. *The inspiratory/expiratory ratio is altered.*
   b. *There is increased likelihood of head colds.*
   c. *Pneumonia poses a greater problem.*
   d. *Artificial respiration must be carried out via the tracheostoma.*
2. *Which of the following bodily functions altered after laryngectomy may correctly be attributed to a change of the fixative function of the larynx?*
   a. *Tendency to constipation*
   b. *Reduced capacity to lift*
   c. *Reduced ability to smell*
   d. *Difficulty in doing pull-ups*
3. *Which of the following activities is* least *compensable after total laryngectomy?*
   a. *Swimming*
   b. *Bathing*
   c. *Tasting food flavors*
   d. *Smoking*

For over a century surgery has been performed to extract larynges. For the quarter century after the first total laryngectomy in 1873, patients were left with open paths up into the hypopharynx and down into the respiratory tree. Aspiration was a constant hazard requiring prosthetic separation of respiration from deglutition routes. Then, in 1894, a surgical tie-off procedure was developed that achieved permanent separation between the hypopharynx and the trachea (Holinger, 1975). Today, these two surgical procedures are at times supplemented by radiation or by radical neck dissection in which the XI cranial nerve and the sternocleidomastoid muscle are sacrificed.

As a result of one or any combination of these procedures, patients immediately face consequences in daily living activities that need to be addressed. Acknowledging the value of preparedness, Terence (*Adelphi*, Act 3, Scene 3), more than 2,100 years ago, observed that the anticipation of consequences is wisdom. This paper reviews these consequences and the means of compensating for or ameliorating their impact.

The function of respiration for laryngeal speakers requires that the respiratory chain from the lip to the larynx to the lung be patent in order to facilitate the metabolic function of the exchange of gases between the atmosphere and capillaries at the alveoli. Pulmonary ventilation through an open chain supersedes the function of deglutition or speech. At rest (e.g., between swallows), the tongue is positioned anteriorly to maintain a patent pharynx. Similarly, pulmonary demands for inhaled oxygen supersede the speech function of exhaling air to initiate phonation. Movement of air through the larynx-to-lip tube then completes the speech function. Aspirated and phonated air is resonated and articulated within these cavities.

In general, the larynx may be thought of as a valve in the lip-to-lung chain that facilitates respiration. As noted by Zemlin (1968), the larynx functions during inhalation to prevent the entrance of foreign substances into the larynx–respiratory tree. During exhalation the laryngeal valve functions in two ways: forcefully expelling foreign substances that threaten to enter the trachea and preventing the escape of air from the lungs. The nonbiologic functions—phonation for speech and emotion—are achieved with minimal valving in the form of vocal fold approximation.

Jackson and Jackson (1937) enumerated nine specific functions of the larynx: respiratory, circulatory, fixative, protective, deglutitive, coughing, expectorative, phonatory, and emotional. Removal of the laryngeal valve by laryngectomy causes alterations in all of these functions. Following is an explanation of how the laryngectomee is able to compensate for these changes.

Respiratory

The larynx functions for respiration in two ways. Passively, it serves as part of the passageway from the atmosphere to the alveoli of the lungs. The second, more significant function is its role in opening or closing the size of that pathway. The glottal area is approximately one-third of the area above and below the larynx (Jackson & Jackson, 1937). After total laryngectomy the area of the stoma generally is greater than the glottal area. When stoma buttons, tracheal buttons, or plastic buttons are inserted, their area usually ranges between 70 and 140 mm. Natvig (1984) reported greater problems in patients whose stomal sizes were less than 80 mm^2. Of greater significance is the absence of delicate valving, unless attempted digitally. Thus there generally is less resistance in the airway after laryngectomy (Brunetti, 1959). Reduced obstruction and resistance in the airway may have several implications. Laryngectomees must be aware that pneumonia can result from failure to breathe deeply enough to utilize the lower lobes. Although some laryngectomees report no significant change in chest cold frequency, many report markedly fewer head colds after laryngectomy (Diedrich & Youngstrom, 1966).

Even when the resistance to airflow is increased by stenosis of the stomal opening or other pulmonary problems, there are no delicate adjustments for partial valving. Ordinarily, removal of one lung by surgery or collapse is not prejudicial. Significant decreases in stoma size may contribute to reduced flow of air, which results in dire consequences both in a diminished intake of oxygen and a disturbance of the acid base in the blood.

Another consequence of the change in pulmonary ventilation relates to the reduced length of the respiratory chain and to the altered resistance at the stoma. By not going through the nose and/or mouth and throat, cold air has less opportunity to be warmed before it enters the lungs. The effect can be painful in severe winters. The temperature of inhaled air may be raised by body heat, either by funneling air from the stoma to the chest and back to the stoma or by covering the neck with a scarf or other clothing. Brunetti (1959) noted that after laryngectomy there is a tendency toward increased airflow rate and for respiratory/expiratory durations to approach parity. Pulmonary ventilation via the tracheostoma allows the laryngectomee to put a clear plastic bag over the head, tied under the chin, with no threat of suffocation as long as the stoma is open. The threat of suffocation during sleep by occlusion of the stoma from blankets or from stomal collapse, appears related to a tendency for the laryngectomee to sleep on his or her back (Diedrich & Youngstrom, 1966; Schutt, 1986). This same threat prevents some laryngectomees from covering the stoma with a turtleneck or a shirt buttoned at the collar. Sucking material into the stoma on inhalation can be minimized by wearing a firm metal or plastic shield between the inner surface of the clothing and the stoma. Threatening suffocation or increased respiratory effort are serious only if they result in stenosis of the tracheal stoma. Such effort could be associated with pleurisy, asthma, emphysema, or other similar respiratory difficulty. The late Hazel Waldron not only had a stoma smaller in size than the fingernail of her small pinkie finger, but on inspiration it shifted from round to an elliptical/oval shape. Because of the potential danger of stenosis, she had her stoma revised surgically. Some laryngectomees continue indefinitely to use a tracheotomy tube or an acrylic button to maintain a patent stoma of adequate size and shape.

Being a neck breather may have positive as well as negative consequences. As mentioned previously, a plastic clothes bag around the neck is not dangerous. If oxygen is needed, however, it must be delivered at the stoma, not to the nose or mouth (Wexler, 1964). If delivered to the mouth/nose, by mask or mouth-to-mouth, air will never reach the lungs. Moreover, in order to perform artificial respiration/resuscitation on non-laryngectomees, the laryngectomee must do so as a stoma-to-mouth activity.

Emergency personnel (e.g., fire, police, airline attendants) need to be aware of and trained in the means of resuscitating the laryngectomee. Precautions for stoma resuscitation for neck breathers have been listed on individual placards and distributed by the International Association of Laryngectomees (IAL) for use in hospital emergency facilities and hospital rooms. The IAL also has prepared wallet-sized cards and windshield stickers containing similar information. In addition, the IAL has encouraged its members to engrave "neck breather" on the back of medical bracelets or necklaces. Finally, it has produced a film, "Three Critical Minutes," made by New Jersey laryngectomees, which is an excellent vehicle for public education.

The laryngectomee is not unlike the small boy who began to cry in Sunday school class when informed of the wondrous ways in which the body functions. His remonstrance was to the effect that God had made him wrong: "My nose runs and my feet smell." Not only does the laryngectomee experience an almost uncontrollable runny nose with a head cold, but he or she also suffers from a diminished sense of olfaction. Of course, this does not prevent others from being aware of the laryngectomee's possible emanation of unpleasant odors, not only from the feet, but from the oral cavity, stoma, and body in general. Thus, the laryngectomee must be especially conscientious about personal hygiene to minimize odors that might be offensive to others (Natvig, 1984).

Separation of the oropharyngeal tube from the respiratory tree means that air no longer passes through the nose, mouth, and throat en route to the lungs. Movement of air through the nose is normally involved in activities such as smelling, sniffing, snoring, and blowing the nose. Movement of air through the mouth is involved in functions of tasting, sipping, smoking, whistling, and blowing musical instruments. Compensation to aid these activities appears to involve the expansion and contraction of the "vocal tract," the oropharyngeal tube.

The ability to smell odors is markedly diminished for most laryngectomees (Johnson, 1960). Smelling does appear to be effected through the nares, rather than through the stoma, as has been suggested at times. An informal canvas I conducted at the Indiana University School of Medicine involved laryngectomees' efforts to smell inhaled stomal air while blindfolded, and with mouth and nose closed. Efforts to identify such distinctive odors as camphor, lemon, garlic, and perfume failed to exceed chance.

Sniffing for a runny nose or for smelling may be facilitated by expansion of the oropharyngeal tube, especially when the lips and one nostril are closed. In 1985 in Atlanta, a man from Jamaica tried this maneuver with his eyes closed. As a mint leaf was passed under his open nostril, he was able to smell and identify mint, his first olfaction in 17 years since laryngectomy. By using this technique in reverse, a laryngectomee may learn to blow his nose by the forceful contraction of an expanded oropharyngeal tube, again facilitated by occlusion of one nostril.

The loss of snoring after laryngectomy may be viewed by the spouse as an asset rather than a liability. Those laryngectomees who elect to smoke after surgery (Kitzing & Toremalm, 1970) may learn to draw in air through the lips into an expanding oropharyngeal tube and to expel smoke via the nose or mouth with a contracting tube. Similarly, a spoon full of soup needing to be cooled need not be held at the stoma. A small amount of air may be expelled from the mouth with modest force by expanding and then contracting the vocal tract. Thus, one may cool soup on a spoon, blow out a lighted match, or inflate a balloon held to the lips (Norgate, 1984). Indeed, a Bronx cheer or "raspberries" may be initiated with the tongue protruded between the lips.

Whistling with the tongue, through the lips or through the teeth, on inhalation or exhalation also requires the expansion and contraction of the oropharyngeal tube. Capacity for generating such positive and negative pressure can be demonstrated by a laryngectomee using an oral manometer (Diedrich & Youngstrom, 1966). The volumes and pressures generated may be sufficient to activate a mouth organ or a recorder, but do not appear great enough to enable a person to play woodwind or brass musical instruments. To play these instruments, the laryngectomee would need to rely on air from the lung, which would allow greater volume and maximal expiratory force. Exhaled air would need to be coupled to the instrument directly from the stoma. More commonly, the laryngectomee funnels air from the lungs into the oral cavity by means of a rubber tube connected to the stoma (Bosone, 1985; Shanks, 1967). Don Schuerman used such a hose to deliver lung air to his mouth so that he could play a trumpet or tuba. For a teacher in West Germany, a seminar was concluded successfully only when he learned to use a rubber hose to divert lung air to the mouth to play his recorder. On the other hand, Red Woodward of Texas, for many years played a recorder held directly in the stoma. Several laryngectomees, including Paul Augenstein, a former IAL president, have played two harmonicas simultaneously—one held at the mouth and one held at the stoma. This is analogous to using a pneumatic artificial larynx whereby air can be shunted via the stoma directly into a mechanical larynx whose source of phonation is a metal reed (WE 2), rubber band (Japanese), or flexible perforated disc (DSP8). Such phonated air must be funneled into the oropharyngeal tube to be resonated and articulated into speech.

Circulatory

The very fluctuations of the laryngeal valve noted in respiration have an impact on blood circulation (Jackson & Jackson, 1937). Thus the pumping action at the capillaries of the alveoli may extend all the way to the heart. After laryngectomy this delicate valving control is removed. I am not aware of any reports, anecdotal or in the scientific literature, of the consequences that total laryngectomy might have on circulatory efficiency.

Fixative

Total valving by adduction of the vocal cords is necessary to permit utilization of expiratory efforts that do not result in loss of air from the lungs. In laryngectomees this function is modified and may affect ability to lift heavy objects, as well as other behaviors involving visceral compression. Thus, the laryngectomee might have difficulty swinging on gymnastic equipment, such as rings, or in doing pull-ups. Even in the absence of prehensile function of the upper limbs, there are times when resisted efforts at pulmonary exhalation are valued, including lifting, parturition, defecation with effort or straining, and even micturation. These behaviors might be accomplished by tensing the rectus abdominis and oblique muscles with the stoma open (Coyne, Stram, Peyton, Klein, & Kressler, 1968); however, a more likely vehicle would be to use stomal blockage by means of a finger.

An Indiana laryngectomee reported that he was able to lift 400 pounds before surgery but only 200 pounds afterward. Lifting may be facilitated by shifting the work to the legs rather than to the trunk. Loss of the laryngeal valve also reduces a mother's ability to assist in childbirth by attempting to exhale with force. Although most female laryngectomees are past the childbearing age, Mary Brink of Minnesota was exceptional as she bore three children after laryngectomy. Pitting expiratory against inspiratory muscles may permit a form of breath holding to aid lifting. At such times, esophageal voice is impaired or precluded. An athletic furniture mover had difficulty shouting a warning when his grip loosened as he was going down stairs. Tendency to constipation may be adequately minimized by suppositories, a mild laxative, or a change of diet with an increase of fiber intake. Finally, it may simply be that laryngectomees cannot lift or compress the abdomen as they did preoperatively without stomal blockage.

Protective

In laryngeal individuals, complete adduction of the laryngeal valve closes the tracheal entrance and enables increased abdominal pressure during forced exhalation. The key role of the larynx in protecting the respiratory tree is the cough reflex, termed the "watchdog of the lung." The mere contact of an object on a vocal fold can cause the adductive forces to spasm. The greater likelihood is that the threat of intrusion of foreign objects may be enough to initiate the cough in order that the larynx not only serve as the barrier but, in fact, repulse the object. This filtering of particles that is shared with the nose and vocal tract may be subsumed by a cover over the tracheal stoma. Failure to occlude the stoma permits the accidental ingress into the lungs of substances as varied as water, food, twigs, bugs, hair, or swabsticks. Moreover, there is a potential danger from fumes containing particles of dust, ink, or chemicals that are suspended in the air.

The filtering of air to remove fine particles can be achieved by a cloth substance, as loose as gauze; a turtleneck sweater/dickey; a buttoned shirt; or polyethylene filters. Use of the E-Z Breathe polyethylene filter permitted its inventor, the late Bob Ferrell, a laryngectomee in Indiana, to continue to ride in his horse patrol. With filtering, a haircut can be obtained without undue risk of inhaling hair particles. The laryngectomee should be alert, however, to hazards from noxious fumes, aerosol sprays, paint, hairspray, powder, or astringent shampoos. A farmer can work without undue risk from dust or insects, a house painter and an employee in a chemical plant can continue to work without undue risk from inhaling fumes, and a printer is able to work in the newspaper press room without undue danger from ink particles in the air.

Filtering of inspired air need not be aseptic or sterile. A polyethylene filter may be replaced or covered by a more cosmetic object. Decorative jewelry, such as items promoted by the laryngectomee club in southern California, crocheted dickeys, and colored scarfs are used frequently by women. Ascots, ties, and turtlenecks are used by men. All are attractive as well as functional for covering the stoma.

Clearly, smoke drawn into the mouth will not transport nicotine into the lungs. Fortunately, few laryngectomees opt to hold a cigarette in the stoma for a diluted drag. Even fewer choose to cut off the tip of a baby bottle nipple to use it as a stomal cigarette holder.

The one foreign substance whose exclusion must be considered separately is water. Showering should proceed with various precautions. One may purchase and use a commercially manufactured shower guard which fits snugly around the neck, yet provides an opening at the bottom to facilitate breathing. Suspending a washcloth from the chin as a drape, or directing the shower spray lower on the chest or on the back are alternatives. Bathing in a tub is safe if the water level does not rise to the chin or above the stoma.

A young mother of four in Kansas continued to water ski after her laryngectomy, with risks reduced by being fitted with a buoyant body-type life preserver designed to hold her higher than normal in the water. A laryngectomized man from South Carolina indulged in scuba diving after having taken the precaution of achieving an airtight fit between the tube tank and his stoma. Swimming activities were reported by 13% of Norwegian laryngectomees (Natvig, 1984). For swimming, as well as for reclining in a bathtub filled with water above the level of the stoma, one may use a LARKEL (LARyngectomee snorKEL). This device, invented by Paul Hauwert of Belgium, includes a flexible rubber tube with an inflatable cuff on one end that expands in the stoma and a rubber mouthpiece on the opposite end. This allows for a connection between the mouth and the trachea. An adaptor can be attached so that the device can be used like a snorkel. A man in Munich used this device for hydrotherapy on his scarred neck while sitting in a full bathtub. Another man used his LARKEL to swim in the pool that was built in his backyard in Louisiana 3 months before his total laryngectomy. Norm Scott, a polio patient from Hawaii, used his device to massage his ego as well as his withered legs by swimming.

Even this device, however, may not be needed. A laryngectomee from Arizona caused spectators some consternation as he first approached the swimming pool, took a big breath, and jammed his forefinger into his stoma before executing a one-armed sailor dive into the pool. He then removed his finger and swam across the pool with no protection over the stoma. I have observed Preben Olsen of Denmark in a pool with no

LARKEL device. He prevented water from entering the lungs by controlling his respiratory system. There is some question as to whether this means merely suspending breathing (contracting neither inspiratory nor expiratory muscles) or using a slight expiratory force to resist the pressure of water at the stomal entrance. Clearly, this technique requires a delicate maneuver that has been learned by only a few. Laryngectomees who fish, hunt birds, or guide small boats over the water are admonished to thrust a hand over the stoma in the event that the boat capsizes. They need not drown.

Deglutitive

The other protective function of the larynx occurs in deglutition. The minor miracle of alternately breathing and swallowing without aspiration or aerophagia is not always appreciated. Following total laryngectomy, there is no longer a need to alternate or synchronize the two functions.

Although it is considered impolite to talk with food in the mouth, laryngeal individuals can talk while eating. Postlaryngectomy, talking while eating is markedly difficult. A laryngectomee using standard esophageal voice becomes a better before-dinner than after-dinner speaker. One option for a laryngectomee at a banquet is to eat heartily, then play back a message previously tape-recorded (Norgate, 1984). Another is to eat before the banquet and forgo food or eat lightly while everyone else enjoys the meal. Incidentally, to gargle after laryngectomy, a person first must deposit air into the esophagus and then let the returning air bubble through liquid placed in the hypopharynx, as demonstrated on videotape by Joe Plotner (Shanks, 1975).

With the surgical tie-off, and in the absence of perforation of the common wall, the aspiration of food or liquid is unlikely. The advent of the tracheoesophageal puncture and prosthesis reminds us, however, that aspiration is indeed a hazard despite the surgical tie-off, whenever the party wall is breached.

Another consequence of the separation of breathing and eating occurs in the hypopharynx. Whereas prelaryngectomy the tongue must be positioned anteriorly to maintain a patent airway, this is no longer needed postlaryngectomy. As noted in a radiographic study by Diedrich and Youngstrom (1966), the tongue often is positioned closer to the posterior pharyngeal wall, without penalty. For esophageal speakers, the dorsum may be positioned higher in the mouth (Noll & Torgerson, 1967). There also is a greater likelihood of chronic pooling of saliva in the hypopharynx, again without penalty or aspiration.

Shipp (1970) reported a change following laryngectomy in the timing of the firing of the inferior pharyngeal constrictor and cricopharyngeal muscles. Before laryngectomy, the two muscles functioned alternately: when one was contracted, the other was relaxed. After surgery, they functioned simultaneously. There may be greater difficulty in retaining and depositing food and liquid in the stomach (Diedrich & Youngstrom, 1966). When tying shoes, bending over at the hips may be accompanied by the loss of gastric juices into the mouth. This implies a loss of tonicity not only at the junction of the pharynx and the esophagus, but also at the cardiac sphincter (Wolfe, Olsen, & Goldenberg, 1971). This reduced tonicity, coupled with the intake of air into the esophagus for esophageal speech, may increase the inadvertent ingestion of air into the stomach. The aerophagia may result in increased flatus, borborygmia, or a "bonus" of esophageal voice (i.e., the true eructation of air by belching). Air thus deposited in the stomach may be irritating to the point of reduced social activity (Natvig, 1984), or it may complicate problems associated with a stomach or duodenal ulcer (King, Fowlks, & Pierson, 1968) or a colostomy. A man from New Jersey noted a need for softer esophageal voice, as well as more sitz baths after colostomy (Wilshaw, 1978).

Deglutition may be impeded in two other ways. Pre- or postoperative radiation therapy tends to alter the flexibility of the swallowing mechanism. This may be accompanied by a drying of the region, with less salivation. A net result may be a need to masticate food into a smaller bolus, and to propel it into the esophagus by means of digital pressure, stroking and pushing down on the anterior neck, or by using liquids to wash down food on the inside. Some laryngectomees benefit from a diet of soft food, such as succulent shrimp scampi (York & Keith, 1983), which may help olfaction. Laryngectomees who have had extensive surgery may use a high-caloric liquid as a diet supplement or as primary diet.

Coughing

The tussive action, coughing, is considered a protective function of the larynx. Following laryngectomy, the expulsion of a foreign object no longer mandates a tight adduction of the tube, with buildup of subglottic pressure to propel the object on vocal cord abduction. Total laryngectomy does not preclude the expulsion of foreign objects. Every laryngectomee knows that coughing does not stop with the removal of the larynx, but that the cough comes from the neck opening, not the mouth. How is the cough achieved? The stoma can be occluded until increased air pressure is generated in the lungs. Without occlusion, the laryngectomee can learn to compress the lungs quickly with ballistic action of the expiratory muscles. Developing this capacity has several implications. Inadvertent expulsion of mucus is reduced by some form of stoma cover. The development of the unresisted cough probably serves to increase the depth of respiration as well as the strength and speed of contraction of muscles of respiration, particularly exhalation muscles (Diedrich & Youngstrom, 1966). A voluntary two-handed cough allows one hand to cover the mouth (for appearance) and one hand to cover the stoma (for business).

The cough function may well increase, especially for the first two years after laryngectomy (Natvig, 1984). Indeed, the cough reflex often is triggered by such stimuli as touching the neck after laryngectomy. A cough may be elicited by the paroxysm of a previous cough. Some laryngectomees find it necessary to maintain minimal physical contact at the neck to reduce the spontaneous cough, whereas others find it helpful to maintain a cover over the stoma which provides for a retention of high-humidity respired air. It may be necessary to exert a willful slowing down of the respiratory/coughing cycle.

The roles of the nose change prior to and after total laryngectomy. The functions of the nose—warming, humidifying, and filtering inhaled air—may be assumed in part by a variety of aids. One is a polyethylene filter. Several laryngectomees have created idiosyncratic devices that allow high humidification of inhaled air by means of a vial of water suspended at the entrance of the stoma. The GIBEK respiration device, made in Sweden, utilizes paper (somewhat resembling a cigarette filter) to retain the humidity of exhaled air for return to the lungs on inspiration. Again, the cough is a crucial variable because it might plug the stoma with mucus. Current reports indicate that coughing is much less likely with use of the filter and the humidifier during pulmonary ventilation, even for persons recently laryngectomized.

Only one laryngeal transplant has been reported. In 1969 Kluyskens successfully transplanted a larynx into a man whose larynx was sacrificed due to carcinoma. Although the man had phonation (somewhat analogous to voice from bilateral paralyzed vocal folds), he was unable to use a cough reflex to protect the respiratory tree (Kluyskens & Ringoir, 1970).

Expectorative

The ability to spit is predicated on the buildup of air pressure behind a bolus or globule of mucus or other object. When air is expelled suddenly, the projectile also is expelled. After laryngectomy there is an absence of forceful pulmonary airflow behind the bolus in the mouth. It is possible, however, to expand and contract the oropharyngeal tube (i.e., vocal tract) to such an extent that a modest force can propel an object forward and past the lips. The compensation presumes the capacity to expand and contract the walls of the pharyngeal and oral cavities. This ability is analogous to building up air pressure to articulate the voiceless consonant /p/ (Shanks & Duguay, 1984). In the absence of the ability to build up significant air pressure, one is reminded of the joke, "I used to be able to spit over my chin; now I spit all over it."

Phonatory

Phonatory compensations are not discussed in this chapter since they are reviewed elsewhere in this book.

Emotional

Jackson and Jackson (1937) noted that vocal cord vibration usually is present during crying, sobbing, moaning, and laughing. Clearly, following laryngectomy, a person's ability to phonate when expressing emotion is severely restricted. The expression of emotion, either positive or negative, is enhanced by audible sound. Suitable options for laughing are available to the laryngectomee: bursts of esophageal tone, bursts of pharyngeal tone, or puffs of stomal expulsion of air. There is no need to limit expressions of amusement to silent laughter or to slapping one's thigh or a table.

The ability to laugh *at* oneself and to find humor in an otherwise serious situation is important. Many laryngectomees have reported with some satisfaction the experience of being approached by a well-intentioned stranger who observes, "My, you certainly do have a bad cold—you'd better take care of your laryngitis." Another favorite report of laryngectomees is that the surgeon cut out snoring when he or she cut out the larynx. Excision of a stentorian stentor usually meets with approval of the spouse. A spouse accustomed to the snoring learns to listen for stoma breathing as a substitute vital sign. Another report of laryngectomees is the prowess of being able to have a prolonged kiss while blowing in the ear of the object of one's affection. The young daughter of a physician reported to her dad when he came home one evening that she had answered the phone for him and had a chance to "talk to a computer." In a similar vein, a woman working at a business was approached by a customer who was trying to reach her on the telephone. The customer complimented her on the remarkable telephone answering service that she maintained in her home. The customer said that not only did the answering service take her message, but it answered the questions that she asked. Clearly, the customer received the benefit of the lady's laryngectomized husband speaking with an electrolarynx. In a similar situation, an ambiguity in telephone conversation prompted a person speaking to a laryngectomee to ask, "Is this an obscene phone call?" Finally, a favorite laryngectomee joke is: "What is the color of a belch?" "Burple!"

The attempt to communicate in the absence of vocal folds requires creative substitute methods. Immediately after the operation, before developing any form of voice, some patients are encouraged to tap on the telephone mouthpiece in an attempt to communicate by telephone. One tap may signify "yes," two taps "no," and three taps "I don't know" or "Please repeat." A desk hand bell can be used in a similar manner. Of course, these systems require that all callers know the code.

In addition to the actual humor involved with speaking, there are ironies that can be at least mildly humorous. Each laryngectomee who attended the annual meeting of the IAL in St. Louis in 1960 was given a door prize: a gilt-edged ashtray. In 1972, the entertainment event of the IAL at Ft. Lauderdale, Florida, involved several hundred laryngectomees sailing on the Atlantic Ocean, singing as a group, while moving to their dinner destination. In 1988, the IAL meeting in Seattle included door prizes of neck pillows that are inflated by blowing air—a difficult feat from the stoma.

CONSEQUENCES OF ADDITIONAL SURGERY/THERAPY ON DAILY LIVING ACTIVITIES

King, Lewis, Weddle, and Fowlks (1973) noted that surgical dissection of the neck to remove lymph nodes and glands is apt to result in reduced sensory function, reduced neck diameter, reduced motor function from muscles available to elevate the ipsilateral arm above the shoulder, and altered blood pressure, especially in the carotid artery and some veins. Physical therapy may facilitate return of arm elevation to the point that labor such as carpentry and barbering may be continued (Schutt, 1986). Reduced blood pressure, rather than reduced resistance to respiration at the stoma, may be responsible for the tendency of some laryngectomees to hyperventilate. Increased sensorineural loss of auditory acuity and marked increase of pressure in internal jugular veins may result from bilateral neck dissection (Gamble & Peterson, 1968).

Neck circumference is reduced following total laryngectomy, and especially after radical neck dissection. Shirt wearers can compensate either by having the collar altered or by moving the top button an appropriate distance. The second button can be sewn over the buttonhole so the shirt always appears buttoned while the wearer has convenient access to the stoma. Another way to provide easy stomal access is to make a vertical opening in the right shirt front. The sides may be bound so it appears to be a pocket. Finally, the tail of the shirt may be used to fashion an ascot-like stoma cover of sartorial splendor.

Although it has been said that laryngectomees no longer hiccup, the fact is that the hiccup is triggered by phrenic nerve contraction of the diaphragm, and may indeed be intractable at times, a singultus. (Incidentally, a hiccup can lead to an inhalation form of air intake into the esophagus for esophageal voice.)

PSYCHOSOCIAL CONSEQUENCES OF LARYNGECTOMY

The effect of the loss of the larynx on the psyche is difficult to assess. The word cancer may conjure up physical suffering and psychological pain (Stoll, 1958). Fortunately, most laryngectomees assume the attitude, "dying of old age doesn't seem so bad when you consider the alternatives." The individual who elects to take his or her own life (Barton, 1965) may have a greater fear of the unknown associated with life on earth than of an afterlife. Part of the psychic disturbance appears to relate to the way in which the laryngectomee thinks he or she will look and sound to society (Gilmore, 1961). The person's attempt to minimize the differences may not be completely successful, but should not deter the laryngectomee who is emotionally healthy. Laryngectomees frequently report a period of postoperative depression and/or withdrawal. As reported anecdotally by William Gargan (1969) in his book *Why Me?* such feelings of depression and isolation may be offset by increased contact with successfully rehabilitated laryngectomees. At the same time it must be acknowledged that these feelings probably are more than the expression of self-pity about the loss of inherent structures and functions of the body.

Interaction with others is a prime factor. Better esophageal speech is achieved when the laryngectomee lives with and relates to other persons rather than when the person lives alone (Diedrich & Youngstrom, 1966). At the same time, the laryngectomee and his or her family may need to learn how to develop new relationships of dependence/independence/interdependence. The laryngectomee should be neither overprotected nor underneeded (Walsh, 1972).

Amputation of the larynx in men has been likened to symbolic castration, a loss of manliness. Laryngectomy may contribute to divorce (Natvig, 1984) or to reduced frequency of sexual intercourse (Meyers, Aarons, Suzuki, & Pilcher, 1980). The spouse who is upset by the mate's hot stomal breath on the neck, may appreciate use of a stoma cover which breaks up the airflow or diverts it away from the stoma. Although radiation associated with laryngectomy may impair sexual performance

(Natvig, 1984), capacity for orgasm should not be affected by laryngectomy itself. A man was atypical in his report of vomit in lieu of orgasm unless he (1) refrained from eating before the act and (2) assumed the missionary posture during intercourse. Healthy marital relationships before laryngectomy often continue to be healthy after laryngectomy (Natvig, 1984). Some laryngectomees, and some counselors (Gonnella, et al., 1978), however, would prefer that sexual relations be included as a topic in counseling (Meyers et al., 1980), perhaps as part of the impact of cancer generally (Stoklosa, Bullard, Rosenbaum, & Rosenbaum, 1980).

The extent to which a person has accepted or reacted appropriately to his or her laryngectomy may be explored in two lines of inquiry. In one line of inquiry, the laryngectomee is asked what he or she did on the night before the laryngectomy. Answers may range from becoming intoxicated, to singing softly, to reciting "Thanatopsis," to praying, to talking to one's family and friends with words of increasing hoarseness. The measure of patients' psychological acceptance of laryngectomy may be gleaned from asking them if, after surgery, they dreamed, and if they appeared in their dreams. If the answer is yes, the question is whether the laryngectomees speak during their dreams, and, if so, whether they use preoperative laryngeal voice or postoperative alaryngeal voice? I have encountered only one laryngectomee who answered "yes" to the question, "Do you speak or talk in your sleep?" Clearly, standard esophageal voice provided the sound.

The psychic defect of laryngectomy is related to the patient's understanding of the surgery and its consequences. Two sources of error may exist: what is said and what is heard. The first has to do with inaccurate or incomplete information provided by the physician (Hoops & Kalfuss, 1969). Even when information is provided, the information may be misunderstood or misinterpreted by the patient. The trauma of dealing with unexpected, major surgery may even preclude comprehension of information given. Duguay (1966) reported that laryngectomees are usually naive and have many misconceptions regarding physiologic functions, including speech, after laryngectomy.

The patient must be approached preoperatively with basic facts regarding the surgery and its consequences. Usually this information is presented orally, but may include some printed data. After surgery the information increases. The amount of additional detail is determined by the patient's questions and initiative.

Among the excellent sources for reading, which should be available to patients, are the following:

Keith, R. L., Shane, H. C., Coates, H. L. C., & Devine, K. D. (1984). *Looking Forward.* New York: Thieme-Stratton.

Lauder, E. (1989–1990). *Self-Help for the Laryngectomee.* San Antonio: Author.

Moss, D. G. (1988). *Why Didn't They Tell Me?* Seattle: Laryngectomee Supply.

Salmon, S. J. (1986). Adjusting to Laryngectomy. *Seminars in Speech and Language, 7,* 67–94.

Walsh, T. F. (1972). Sound the Way for Laryngectomees. *Patient Care, 6,* 58–89.

A fine film, produced by the American Cancer Society, is "To Speak Again." Anecdotal reports in local newspapers and periodicals, by or about laryngectomees, also help to present information (see Salmon, 1986, listed above). An outstanding report about a laryngectomized couple, Mabel and Ray Disinger, was written by Perkins (1978).

The IAL has a network of over 300 local clubs. Representatives also gather annually. The clubs are especially helpful as vehicles for sharing information, group discussions of common concerns, and mutual support. Some of the local clubs maintain visitor programs in which a member (often with the spouse) calls on recently operated persons. The visitor is trained to answer questions orally and to distribute pamphlets.

At each annual meeting of the IAL, about 5 hr are devoted to speech therapy. Beginning or problem speakers may require individual counsel, whereas good or advanced speakers may benefit from group therapy. For more than a decade beginning in the mid-1970s, I was privileged to conduct this advanced class. We allocated 4 hr to aspects of speech improvement. The final hour focused on "teaching tips" and consequences of total laryngectomy. At times I referred to it as ADL/ADL (Activities of Daily Living/After Dis Laryngectomy). In a group discussion setting, many laryngectomees volunteer to comment on their perceptions and experiences. Over 3 decades, I have observed shifts in attitudes regarding the impact of total laryngectomy. The nature of comments and attitudes of physiologic change after surgery indicates that the evolution has occurred as follows:

1. Assume/expect minimal change of physiology after laryngectomy.
2. Assert/predict minimal change of physiology after laryngectomy.
3. Identify specific changes or losses of physiologic function after laryngectomy.
4. Discuss changes of physiology in terms of compensations.

A review of these factors signals a move from more negative to more positive attitudes. Such a move is significant. Is the glass half empty or half full? Is there only loss or is there some gain and compensation?

REFERENCES

Barton, R. T. (1965). Life after laryngectomy. *Laryngoscope, 75*, 508–515.

Bosone, Z. T. (1989–1990). A simple device for smelling and nose blowing after laryngectomy. In E. Lauder (Ed.), *Self-help for the laryngectomee* (pp. 83–93), San Antonio: Author.

Brunetti, F., Jr. (1959). Observations of the respiratory dynamic in laryngectomized patients. *Acta Otolaryngologica* (Stockholm), *50*, 334–343.

Coyne, J. M., Stram, J. R., Peyton, O. D., Klein, G. A., & Kressler, J. F. (1968). The laryngectomee and lifting. *Archives of Otolaryngology, 88*, 80–83.

Diedrich, W. M., & Youngstrom, K. A. (1966). *Alaryngeal speech.* Springfield, IL: Charles C. Thomas.

Duguay, M. J. (1966). Preoperative ideas of speech after laryngectomy. *Archives of Otolaryngology, 83*, 69–72.

Gamble, J. E., & Peterson, E. (1968). The effect of increased venous pressure on hearing. *Journal of the Southern Medical Association, 61*, 580–584.

Gargan, W. (1969). *Why me?* New York: Doubleday.

Gilmore, S. I. (1961). Rehabilitation after laryngectomy. *American Journal of Nursing, 61*, 86–89.

Gonnella, C., Parker, D., Hollender, J., Lowell, G., Peterson, P., & Miller, S. (1978). *Normative criteria for cancer rehabilitation* (Rehabilitation Research Monograph Series No. 1). Atlanta: Emory University.

Holinger, P. H. (1975). A century of progress in laryngectomies in the northern hemisphere. *Laryngoscope, 85*, 322–332.

Hoops, H. R., & Kalfuss, H. A. (1969, July). *Counseling the laryngectomee: A study of the surgeon's approach.* Paper presented at the ninth IAL Voice Institute, Pittsburg.

Jackson, C., & Jackson, C. L. (1937). *The larynx and its diseases.* Philadelphia: Saunders.

Johnson, C. L. (1960). A survey of laryngectomee patients in Veterans Administration Hospitals. *Archives of Otolaryngology, 72*, 768–773.

King, P. S., Fowlks, E. W., & Pierson, G. A. (1968). Rehabilitation and adaptation of laryngectomy patients. *American Journal of Physical Medicine, 47*, 192–203.

King, P. S., Lewis, F. R., Weddle, J. L., & Fowlks, E. W. (1973). Effect of radical neck dissection on total rehabilitation of the laryngectomee. *American Journal of Physical Medicine, 52*, 1–16.

Kitzing, P., & Toremalm, N. G. (1970). The situation of the laryngectomized patient. *Acta Otolaryngologica, 263*, 119–123.

Kluyskens, P., & Ringoir, S. (1970). Follow-up of a human larynx transplantation. *Laryngoscope, 80*, 1244–1250.

Meyers, A. D., Aarons, B., Suzuki, B., & Pilcher, L. (1980). Sexual behavior following laryngectomy. *Ear, Nose and Throat Journal, 59*, 327–329.

Natvig, K. (1984). Laryngectomees in Norway. Study #5: Problems in every day life. *Journal of Otolaryngologica, 13*, 15–22.

Noll, J. D., & Torgerson, J. K. (1967). A cinefluorographic observation of the tongue in esophageal speakers. *Folia Phoniatrica, 19*, 343–350.

Norgate, S. (1984). *Laryngectomy is not a tragedy.* Edinburgh: Churchill Livingstone.

Perkins, W. H. (1978). Laryngectomy. In W. H. Perkins (Ed.), *Human perspectives in speech and language disorders* (pp. 238–257). St. Louis: Mosby.

Schutt, A. H. (1986). Physical and occupational therapy for the patient with laryngectomy: Why and what for? In R. L. Keith & F. L. Darley (Eds.), *Laryngectomee rehabilitation* (2nd ed., pp. 295–308). Austin, TX: PRO-ED.

Shanks, J. C. (1967). Advantages in the use of esophageal speech by a laryngectomee. *Laryngoscope, 77,* 239–243.

Shanks, J. C. (1975). *Abilities of laryngectomees* [Videotape]. Indianapolis: Medical Education Resources Program.

Shanks, J. C., & Duguay, M. J. (1984). Voice remediation and the teaching of alaryngeal speech. In S. Dickson (Ed.), *Communication disorders: Remedial principles and practices* (2nd ed., pp. 275–287). Glenview, IL: Scott Foresman.

Shipp, T. (1970). EMG of pharyngoesophageal musculature during alaryngeal voice production. *Journal of Speech Hearing Research, 13,* 184–192.

Stoklosa, J. M., Bullard, D. G., Rosenbaum, E. W., & Rosenbaum, I. R. (1980). Sexuality and cancer. In *A comprehensive guide for cancer patients and their families* (pp. 6-1 to 6-18). Palo Alto: Bull Publishing.

Stoll, B. (1958). Psychological factors determining the success or failure of the rehabilitation program of laryngectomized patients. *Annals of Otology, Rhinology and Laryngology, 67,* 550–557.

Walsh, T. F. (1972). Sound the way for laryngectomees. *Patient Care, 6,* 58–89.

Wexler, D. (1964). Resuscitation for neck breathers. *With New York Firemen, 25*(4), 8–11.

Wilshaw, J. (1978). *After the laryngectomy: A post-operative orientation.* Danville, IL: Interstate Printers and Publishers.

Wolfe, R. D., Olsen, J. E., & Goldenberg, D. B. (1971). Rehabilitation of the laryngectomee: The role of the distal esophageal sphincter. *Laryngoscope, 81,* 1971–1978.

York, J., & Keith, R. L. (1983). Personal health adjustments following laryngectomy, *HELP employ laryngectomized persons.* [Videotape No. 5]. Indianapolis: Medical Education Resources Program.

Zemlin, W. R. (1968). *Speech and hearing science.* Englewood Cliffs, NJ: Prentice-Hall.

CHAPTER 12

Conducting Alaryngeal Speech Rehabilitation Workshops

Robert L. Keith

Keith provides general guidelines for conducting a successful rehabilitation workshop. He supplies details on every aspect of planning from selection of staff to obtaining adequate funding. He discusses possible pitfalls, as well as the personal and professional rewards associated with such a responsibility.

Study Questions

1. *What are three criteria that one should consider in staff selection?*
2. *What are the important aspects of site selection for the workshop?*
3. *How important are budgetary considerations when planning a meeting? Explain your answer.*

A prescription for a successful alaryngeal speech rehabilitation meeting cannot be written, and a paper covering every detail cannot be prepared. General guidelines can be given, however. Then practical knowledge and common sense can be applied in planning and organizing. Although organization of meetings can require a committee, I have never used one. I have found that the efficiency of a committee is inversely proportional to the number of participants and the time spent on deliberations. In other words, I believe that the more I can handle myself, the better informed I will be and the less time I will be involved in total planning. Instead of a committee, I prefer having a secretary and a codirector. The codirector assumes responsibilities for local arrangements and can be of utmost assistance if the meeting is held in another city. The codirector should be a professional with an interest in the area of laryngectomee rehabilitation.

An overview is provided, followed by additional discussion that I hope will be helpful. If you are experienced at arranging conferences, the overview may be sufficient.

APPROACHES TO SUCCESSFUL MEETINGS

Initial planning is probably the most important ingredient for a successful workshop. Some questions must be addressed in determining the purpose for the meeting:

1. What actually is the need?
2. How widespread is the need?
3. Is it a short-term need?
4. Who is in need?
5. What is the scope of need?
6. What is the background of those who have the need?
7. What is the educational background of the group?
8. How can one effectively develop a program to meet needs of participants with different backgrounds and educational experience:
   a. Physicians
   b. Speech pathologists
   c. Social workers
   d. Nurses
   e. Laryngectomees
   f. Significant others

When the initial needs are identified, the task is to decide where and how these needs can be met. Factors to consider include the following:

1. Location
2. Meeting room facilities, lecture halls
3. Audiovisual facilities
4. Housing facilities that are comfortable yet inexpensive
5. Eating facilities
6. Available calendar dates that do not conflict with other scheduled conferences
7. Recreational facilities
8. Transportation
9. Cooperation of some community service organization or national agency

STAFF SELECTION

A tentative selection of a staff needs to be considered. This staff needs flexibility in their abilities and experience; they need to complement each other, work together, and be able to fill in for each other if illnesses or other problems occur. This staff should have the ability to cover the areas of the specialties being presented. The authorities in the field are essential; however, these authorities should not all have the same special interest, be from the same area of the country, or be of the same age. There needs to be a flavor of what occurs in different geographical areas around the country and young staff members to replace older staff as retirement takes place or ratings indicate change is necessary. I suggest using some local people, but also having a core group to provide continuity.

Anticipate possible disasters. What will you do if a speaker cancels within 48 hr of scheduled presentation time? Calm down, do not push the panic button! *STOP, THINK, ACT.* What options do you have?

1. Cancel that presentation.
2. Find a fill-in from outside.
3. Use another faculty member to discuss the topic.
4. Form a panel of attending faculty to present their views on the topic and to conduct a question session.

PROGRAM DEVELOPMENT

Once you have a tentative staff, begin to develop a tentative program to see if all needs are being met. Needless to say, every need cannot be met, as needs are everchanging, and each region or medical institution has different needs, but you need to encompass a broad spectrum so that all will profit. The staff can assist with program planning, as each person should be requested to suggest the topics he or she can and will present.

TRAVEL ARRANGEMENTS

Making travel arrangements is always a delight because it means you are going someplace and can look forward to a wonderful trip if you plan ahead. One important aspect is to identify a travel agent with whom you can work easily. You need to explain your needs and determine what the agent can offer. Generally you can arrange to use one airline and receive a discount on all tickets, or you will be given a few free tickets for a specified number of tickets sold. If you prefer, you may contact an airline directly. The one that is convenient for the largest number of participants should be contacted. Usually prices are quite similar, but it is worthwhile to check with at least two airlines.

MEETING PLACE

The location of the meeting needs to be considered with great care. The following questions are important:

1. How will the staff of the hotel (or other facility) work with you?
2. Will the hotel give you a written agreement?
3. What are costs for lecture halls?
4. What are costs for audiovisual equipment?
5. Does the hotel offer any free services, such as welcoming cocktails, free guest room for the director, or one free room per specified number of hotel registrants?
6. Do you get a better rate if you meet during certain times of the year?
7. Do you get a better rate at certain times of the week? Many hotels are cheaper if a weekend is used; others are cheaper if used midweek.
8. For meal functions, how far in advance must notification of the number of people be given? What leeway are you given on the number of guaranteed dinners? Some institutions require 48 hr advanced guarantee with an estimate at 72 hr, but usually they are prepared to serve 5% to 7% over the guaranteed number. Never give the actual number of tickets sold. For example, if you have sold 100 tickets, and the hotel has a 7% flexibility, then guarantee for only 95. You are covered for the tickets sold, and if some do not show up you will have a little cushion to meet other small costs.
9. Does the meal price include taxes and gratuities?

10. What other social amenities will the hotel give or allow at meal functions?
    a. Centerpieces
    b. Piano
    c. Microphone at speaker's stand
    d. Placecards for tables
    e. If a buffet, allow setup so people may return for seconds
11. If wine is to be served with the meal, the type, brand, and price must be decided beforehand, or you could end up with an expense for which you are not prepared. You can plan for one glass per guest or one carafe per table. Never allow for free-flowing alcohol unless you have an unlimited budget. The best approach is to have a cash bar before the meal function. Even then you must check on the cost. Many places have a minimum charge for the bar; that is, if so many dollars worth are sold in a specific time you have no additional charge. If the bar does not sell enough, you pay so much per hour. You may be able to come to some reasonable figure with the agency. Be sure your agreement is in writing. Never rely on only a verbal commitment.

FUNDING

Where does funding come from and how do you get it? Funding may be arranged through the International Association of Laryngectomees (IAL) or a New Voice Club. Part of it may come from the American Cancer Society (local, state, or national). It is also possible to get some additional funding from the IAL Auxiliary, but this should be considered an emergency fund.

Funding should be requested from the IAL, New Voice Club, or ACS treasurer with copies of the request going to the clubs' executive directors, service officers, or presidents. Your moneys can be obtained at various times as funding is needed. The director of the workshop would normally write all checks, but arrangements should be made so that the codirector is able to write checks in case of an emergency.

Some local funding may be available to underwrite social events, printing, and so forth. Check with local service organizations.

An interest-paying checking account in the name of the workshop should be established. The account should have the director's and a cosigner's (e.g., the codirector's) signatures. Be sure to secure the tax-exempt number of the sponsoring organization(s).

I have indirectly talked about the budget. Now let us look closely at costs. Although there can be hidden expenses, the following are the major ones:

1. Staff
   a. Travel
   b. Honorariums
   c. Per diem
2. Advertising
3. Telephone calls
4. Postage
5. Audiovisual equipment
6. Coffee breaks
7. Meal functions (continental breakfast, banquet, buffet)
8. Secretarial service
9. Entertainment
10. Duplication of materials (sometimes a speaker will bring only one copy of his or her handouts and expect that sufficient copies will be made at the meeting place)
11. Scholarships or other travel assistance
12. Printing of the program
13. Special instrumentation
14. Costs associated with offering continuing education credits

If the above items are considered at the going rate, you can come within 5% to 10% of the estimated budget. Look for volunteer services and other ways to reduce costs. Assistance can come in many forms:

1. Your local place of employment
2. Local service agencies
3. Support groups
4. State organizations in that specialty
5. National organizations
6. Auxiliary groups
7. Pharmacy companies
8. Book publishers
9. Purchase all items for coffee breaks from one supplier (discounts are often allowed for volume buying)
10. Donations of instruments and other materials. Contact the appropriate company by a personal letter explaining the function of the workshop. When seeking the help of an organization, explain what you need from them, how it will be used, what geographic areas are represented by the audience, and how many people will be attending. Offer to supply any other information they may request. If possible, always write to a specific individual and not simply to the company itself. Your success will be greater if you have a contact person. It is important to follow up after the meeting. Express your appreciation and provide general information concerning the

outcome of the meeting. State the number who attended and the geographical areas represented. Companies appreciate this because they then know who was exposed to their advertising and can estimate the effectiveness. Consequently, they are more likely to contribute to a similar event in the future.

Do not forget the chamber of commerce in the meeting city. The chamber can assist in many ways with free maps and information about the city (things to do, restaurants, etc.).

Take bids for printing of announcements and programs, or contact printers to see whether any will volunteer to print free or at reduced prices. Some organizations that hire the handicapped will do printing jobs very reasonably if they are in need of projects. Keep in mind that they often need more time to accomplish the task, so start early!

DISPLAYS

Free display materials should be requested from companies that manufacture products used by attendees. Acknowledge receipt and extend appropriate thanks for the generous giving of free display materials. Display them appropriately, but do not favor one company over another. You must remain nonjudgmental.

Publishing companies often are willing to send free literature about available books on the subject and to furnish a complementary book for exhibit. If this is an annual meeting, request permission to keep the book for future displays. If this workshop is a one-time meeting, have a book sale the last day. If there are only a couple of books to exhibit, have a drawing and give them away. Acknowledge to the publishing company receipt of the literature and the book(s).

If particular books or booklets are frequently used by professionals interested in alaryngeal speech, notify the participants in advance that these publications will be available and list the price of each. Have the participants preorder so that you know how many of each publication to have available. Quantity orders are generally a little cheaper than single copy orders. Confirm this with the publisher.

Do you want an exhibit? You must decide if you have space. Do you want a commercial exhibit, or would you rather not have company representatives? You may want materials and books displayed so that each participant can look at and handle them without feeling any obligation to a sales representative. Both approaches have merit. I prefer having only an exhibit. Often it is not feasible for company representatives to be present because the limited audience does not offer enough exposure.

If you decide to have only an exhibit area, decide on the materials you want to display. Write to each company explaining what you want, why, and how it will be used. Send a copy of the program and guarantee that the materials will be returned by a specific date. Be sure to acknowledge receipt and to express your appreciation. Return all loaned materials promptly. Most companies will cooperate very well. I find this approach allows people the freedom to look at the displays whenever they have free time between sessions. It also allows the director the opportunity to select materials that are appropriate for this type of meeting.

BREAKS AND TIME OFF

Coffee breaks are an essential part of a meeting as they rejuvenate the mind. What will you serve? It depends on a number of factors. How much money do you have to spend? How available is the coffee? How much time can be allotted? Another consideration is whether a continental breakfast is served at the hotel and included as part of the room rate. If so, then serve coffee and decaffeinated coffee, tea, and maybe fresh fruit at the morning break. In the afternoon, serve coffee, tea, soft drinks, and maybe cookies. Food is not necessary at both coffee breaks, but it should be served at least once. This helps to add some warmth, allow for conversation, and encourage socialization that can really enhance communication, building of professional relationships, and a feeling of a successful workshop.

Time off needs to be scheduled. Since most people travel from a distance and are not familiar with the community, arrange a group tour to a community highlight, or provide a listing of possible tours and places of interest. This tour is generally offered as an optional activity and should be paid for separately unless you include this in a registration fee. Having done it both ways, I believe that the freedom of choice is best, although this does require more work on the director's part.

CONTINUING EDUCATION UNITS

With the present need for continuing education credits, make certain this option is available for those participants who desire it. Also, let them know in advance what the fee will be.

This makes for a bit more paperwork, and sometimes I wonder if it is worthwhile. I think so. At this stage of our profession, people look for programs with continuing education credits, so your attendance may be greater because you offer them.

If the sponsoring organization is approved by American Speech–Language–Hearing Association (ASHA), you need only contact ASHA and complete the appropriate form for continuing education units. Be sure to do this early so you can advertise as such. If your sponsoring organization is not approved, then contact your state speech and hearing association or a university. You can have the credits offered through them for a small fee, which is easier than becoming a certified sponsoring organization. Also, the other organization will handle most of the paperwork.

HANDOUTS AND AUDIOVISUAL AIDS

Your staff is the backbone of the workshop. Let them know in advance the program schedule and their specific lecture topics and times. Request their needs for audiovisual aids so you are not caught without a piece of equipment necessary to make the lecture outstanding. Handouts should be encouraged, but they are best placed in a packet and handed out at registration. The speaker should either furnish ample copies or send the original at least 6 weeks in advance for reproduction. If you offer to make copies for the staff, be sure that this cost is planned in the budget. Encourage readable slides. Slide presentations are important, but printed material presented on slides should be limited. If it is used at all, encourage printing that is large enough to be read by those sitting in the back rows.

ADVERTISING

Advertising is important, but where and how is probably most important. One of the most effective ways is via word of mouth. According to a survey taken at two meetings I directed, 75% heard about the workshops by word of mouth. It is unfortunate that we cannot all be on street corners and shout the word! Instead, we need to reach every media that is appropriate, so that someone else can spread the word for us. The most important publications to use are ASHA's Calendar of Events, IAL's Newsletter, and every New Voice Club newsletter. Also, a notice should be sent to every state Speech–Language–Hearing Association.

SUMMARY EVALUATION

A summary evaluation needs to be prepared. It should include an overview of pertinent information, number of attendees, the number of participants accepted and the number rejected, names of speakers, geographical areas where advertised, total number of phone calls made during the planning year, any other similar information, and a summary of the overall evaluation done by the attendees.

The participants should evaluate each speaker, the organization of the meeting, the site, the food, coffee breaks, facilities, advertising, and future needs. The participants can give a more objective evaluation than the director. A director too often perceives what he or she wants to perceive, when actually the needs may not have been met. On the other hand, the director may find that the needs of the group have been met beyond all expectations. The comments received from those in attendance help direct future planning in the area. One can correct weaknesses and maintain strengths.

Where appropriate, final summaries should go to all organizations financially involved. Each staff member should receive his or her own evaluation. The general summary is needed primarily by the director and codirector(s) for future planning.

I suggest that the director perform a final budget analysis and pay all bills. He or she should receive compensation for all expenses and an honorarium to compensate for time away from work. Also, I would advise refunding any money left over to supporting agencies.

FORMULA FOR PROGRAM FORMAT

The formula for a successful program is a ratio of 5:3—five lectures and three clinical experiences daily. First and foremost is the didactic. For every 5 hr of lecture presentation, there should be 2 hr of clinical practice and 1 hr of group discussion. Each supervisory staff member should not be assigned more than 10 pairs of one laryngectomee and one speech pathologist. During a week-long workshop, each staff member should be expected to supervise two therapy sessions and one rap session each day. He or she could probably present 8 to 10 lectures during the meeting, if there are dual tracks, one for professionals and one for laryngectomees and significant others.

COMPLAINTS

People are quick to complain about all possible things:

- Can't hear
- Too hot, too cold
- Someone forgot to bathe
- Someone wears too much perfume
- Someone is always late

- Not enough bathrooms at coffee breaks
- Cannot stand to be working with someone
- Cannot understand because of accent
- Do not like jokes that are told
- Do not like off-colored jokes
- Weather not cooperative
- Travel too difficult
- Occupants in next room noisy
- Some people are clannish and do not associate with others
- Not enough special diets
- Start later in day
- Cut lecture time
- Add more lectures
- More breaks
- Cannot stand any smoking
- Too costly
- Better places to meet
- Cheaper places to meet
- Arrange for church services

The list could go on, and actually sometimes you get a good laugh out of it all. Someone wrote, "May I bring my dog? He's my best friend!"

EMERGENCIES

Emergencies always occur. What type? Who knows? Cardiac arrest, food stuck in esophagus, diabetic reaction, sprained ankles, recurrences of tumors, deaths in family, insect bites, mild stroke, forgetting medication, angry spouses, threatening phone calls, loss of personal items, money lost, special dietary needs, stoma occlusion, migraine headaches, alcoholism. The list could go on. Over the years these have all occurred. First and foremost, be prepared!

1. Have emergency numbers.
    a. Police
    b. Doctor
    c. Hospital
    d. Hotel
    e. Church list
2. Be aware of special abilities within your staff for dealing with emergencies.
3. Follow emergencies through with your utmost attention. This is important; the people are away from home, and you may be their only friend.

DIRECTOR AND CODIRECTOR

The director needs to have total control of directing and planning the workshop without the necessity of meeting with committees to make decisions. If assistance is needed, advice can be obtained from lecturing staff members or a member of the Speech Standards Committee of the IAL, New Voice Club, or ACS. Also, the director should be the person responsible for all advertising, which must begin about a year in advance.

To obtain an even geographic balance, the director should be responsible for accepting all speech pathologists and laryngectomees. The acceptance for scholarships should be done at the time applications are received. If a person requests a scholarship, he or she should be requested to provide the following information: his or her approximate income and cost of travel to the workshop. Speech pathologists should be asked if their employers are giving financial assistance to attend the institute.

Being the director of a workshop is short of glory but full of personal satisfaction. People are quick to complain but slow to praise, so do not look for very many compliments. Have a barrel of "energy pills," for you need to run on high. Know what is going on so you are abreast of happenings. Keep your lines of communication open with your staff. They are the backbone of the workshop and know of problems early on. It is easier to handle problems before they are full-blown.

Somewhere along the way, many rough, bumpy, treacherous roads appear, along with dead ends, and you would like to forget them. Look at it this way. This is just another wonderful challenge in your professional growth. You do not have to repeat the act if you do not like it, but do your best. That is all one can ask.

Have I learned anything over the years as director of laryngectomee workshops and IAL voice institutes? I had no idea of the work involved. If I had not been so naive for the first laryngectomee seminar, I wonder if I would have gone through with it. Yes, absolutely! It is a service that is needed and continues to be needed. Remember, your workshop staff can be of tremendous assistance in finalizing the program. They are more or less your committee, except you have the final decision. Would I change many things? By all means, no. I personally would not even attempt to run a seminar or institute by establishing a whole formal committee. It is too time-consuming. During my first seminar, three of us worked on planning and organization. We met four times during the year. For the second and succeeding years there have been only two of us. Believe me, use of the telephone is a necessity.

My final advice to anyone conducting a workshop is to have an understanding family. Be prepared to devote many hours prior to and during the actual meeting times. If the workshop is in your home town, you may not even get home. Involve the family if you can in order to see them, or for them to see you and realize you are working very hard.

You will be rewarded with the personal satisfaction of a job well done for the betterment of mankind.

Author Index

Subject Index

Vocal range, in refinement program of esophageal speech training, 85–86

Vocational factors. *See* Occupational factors

Voice parameters
  of artificial larynx speech, 178, 182
  in esophageal speech, 177, 178
  in refinement program of esophageal speech training, 84–86

Voice prothesis. *See also* Prostheses
  insertion of, 121–122
  low-pressure or low-resistance voice prosthesis, 125–126
  selection of optimal prosthesis type, 124–125

Voiced sounds, in esophageal speech, 18–19

Voiceless sounds, in esophageal speech, 18

Vowels, in esophageal speech, 19–20

Western Electric #5, 30, 32, 42

Workshops
  advertising for, 267
  approaches to successful meetings, 260–261
  breaks and time off, 266
  complaints, 268–269
  Continuing Education Units for, 266–267
  director and codirector of, 270–271
  displays, 265–266
  emergencies, 269
  formula for program format, 268
  funding for, 263–265
  handouts and audiovisual aids, 267
  meeting place, 262–263
  program development of, 261–262
  staff selection for, 261
  summary evaluation of, 267–268
  travel arrangements for, 262